GUIDE TO
DIAGNOSTIC PROCEDURES

FOURTH EDITION

GUIDE TO DIAGNOSTIC PROCEDURES

RUTH M. FRENCH

Associate Dean
Professor of Medical Laboratory Sciences
School of Associated Medical Sciences
College of Medicine
University of Illinois Medical Center, Chicago

McGRAW-HILL BOOK COMPANY

A Blakiston Publication

New York St. Louis San Francisco Auckland Düsseldorf
Johannesburg Kuala Lumpur London Mexico
Montreal New Delhi Panama Paris São Paulo
Singapore Sydney Tokyo Toronto

GUIDE TO DIAGNOSTIC PROCEDURES

1234567890MUMU798765

This book was set in Theme by Allen Wayne Technical Corp. The
editors were Cathy Dilworth and Shelly Levine Langman; the cover
was done by Scott Chelius; the production supervisor was Charles
Hess.
The Murray Printing Company was printer and binder.

NOTICE

Medicine is an ever-changing science. As new research and
clinical experience broaden our knowledge, changes in treatment
and drug therapy are required. The editors and the publisher of this
work have made every effort to ensure that the drug dosage
schedules herein are accurate and in accord with the standards
accepted at the time of publication. The reader is advised, however,
to check the product information sheet included in the package of
each drug he plans to administer to be certain that changes have
not been made in the recommended dose or in the contraindications
for administration. This recommendation is of particular importance in regard to new or infrequently used drugs.

Library of Congress Cataloging in Publication Data

French, Ruth M
    Guide to diagnostic procedures.

    "A Blakiston publication."
    First-3d ed. published under title: Nurse's guide to
diagnostic procedures.
    Includes bibliographies and index.
    1. Diagnosis. 2. Medicine, Clinical—Laboratory
manuals. I. Title. [DNLM: 1. Diagnosis, Laboratory—
Nursing texts. QY4 F875n]
RB37.F79 1975   616.07'5   75-6841
ISBN 0-07-022141-3
ISBN 0-07-022140-5 pbk.

CONTENTS

PREFACE

In response to many suggestions, this fourth edition of "The Nurse's Guide to Diagnostic Procedures" has been titled "Guide to Diagnostic Procedures" in recognition of the fact that the previous editions have been used by a variety of health-care professionals.

Any health-care professional looking over developments in the past few decades cannot help being impressed by the increasing depth of detailed understanding of the multiple factors contributing to the often delicate balance between health and susceptibility to, or actual, pathology. The rapidity with which the esoterica of research are translated into daily practice is just as impressive. Significant elements of each of these characteristics are the products of sophisticated instrumentation and equally sophisticated professional staff personnel who perform the diagnostic procedures. A natural tendency is toward specialization. Yet, the more specialized we health professionals become, the more we must work together if we are to counterbalance fragmentation in diagnosis and treatment.

Cooperation among health-services personnel increases the quality of care and enhances each person's own unique services. As in any area of life, cooperation finds its strength in understanding. It is this goal of cooperation, achieved by understanding, that I have endeavored to reach with this book. The major part of "Guide to Diagnostic Procedures" is concerned with explanations of fundamental principles, definitions of the more common terms associated with diagnosis, the role of the nurse in each of the diagnostic tests, and interpretation of results. The diagnostic procedures themselves have been described in the least amount of detail necessary to provide the framework for understanding the demands made upon all concerned: the patient, health professionals assisting the departments that provide diagnostic services, and the personnel of those departments.

In addition to serving the above goal, the text can be used as a reference for patient education. The health professional is increasingly called upon to explain diagnostic procedures and interpretations to patients and to allow them to take part in making decisions about their own bodies. This role is, first, a product of the public's increasing sophistication about things medical and of the layman's desire to know what is being done. Secondly, the force of law and mores demands that the patient's right to informed consent be honored. This edition is, therefore, like the previous editions, expected to assist health professionals in meeting this responsibility.

No technical book is completely the original work of its author. In recognition of this, I would like to express my appreciation to the authors and publishers whose material I have drawn upon for their permission to share their work. Many people have had a hand in the completion of this edition, through their suggestions and their sharing of insights into the needs to be met by such a text. Although they are too numerous to mention by name, I wish to acknowledge their contributions with my thanks.

Ruth M. French

GUIDE TO
DIAGNOSTIC PROCEDURES

ONE

DIMENSIONS OF QUALITY

The commitment of anyone serving in the health professions must be to the principle that the "patient is the central imperative."[1] He or she is our whole reason for the very fact that there are health professions. Too often that commitment can become alloyed by natural human tendencies toward self-concern. However, one can use even that self-concern in a positive way if its energies are channeled into motivation to be the best possible steward of one's knowledge, skill, and judgment. With such an approach to one's work, benefits to the patients are assured, and there is satisfaction in achievement that serves the psychologic needs each of us has.

There are those who wonder how a medical technologist can keep a fresh concern for the patient as a person when contacts

[1] Mary K. Mullane, Ph.D., Dean Emeritus, College of Nursing, University of Illinois at the Medical Center.

1

with the patient are limited. (Indeed, the technologist may not even see patients on a daily basis.) One of the regular reminders is the realization that the data being provided by the medical laboratory are particularly important because they constitute the bulk of the quantitative, objective information about the patient. This characteristic results in a significant weight of responsibility which makes the technologist keenly conscious of her duty to the patient as a person. Thus, a tube of blood is not, in her mind, a disconnected entity but an extension of the patient—a life in her hands.

The patient puts his faith in us, more often than not, blindly. He seldom has the opportunity to see what is being done with specimens and, even if he did, would not be able to judge the quality of the work more than superficially. Honoring that faith is our responsibility.

Proper use of the diagnostic services of the laboratory and radiology departments is of utmost importance if the patient's needs are to be maximally met with a minimum of discomfort, expense, and time. This calls for planning, not only on the part of the physician in ordering appropriate procedures and putting the information gained into the diagnostic process, but also on the part of those involved in patient care so that scheduling is accomplished efficiently and effectively.

A term common to many different contexts is "routine." The usual connotation when applied to an activity is that it is repetitive and dull. In the medical laboratory, however, it is much more meaningful. It means that a test is so important to so many patients that it is frequently requested. For example, routine tests such as the blood count and urinalysis can reflect evidence of unsuspected disease and thus can redirect diagnostic investigation. The purpose of this chapter is to discuss some of the elements of the medical laboratory routines which express the commitment to the patient as the central imperative. In addition, there are routine concepts which must be understood by all who use the data if the tests are to be given appropriate value in the diagnostic or treatment processes.

UNITS OF MEASUREMENT

Reports of laboratory tests are made in a variety of terms, depending on the nature of the compound or element being evaluated. The meanings of these terms are discussed in order to clarify their significance and interpretation. Precise measurements are expressed with the metric system. Table 1-1 presents the metric system nomenclature and relationships between the units in magnitude.

TABLE 1-1   METRIC SYSTEM MEASUREMENTS

Unit	Abbreviation	Metric equivalent	Nonmetric equivalent
Length			
Meter	m		39.37 in.
Centimeter	cm	1/100 m	
Millimeter	mm	1/1,000 m	
Micron	μ	10^{-6} m, 10^{-3} m,	
Nanometer	nm	10^{-9} m	
Weight			
Kilogram	kg		2.205 lb
Gram	g	1/1,000 kg	453.6 g = 1 lb
Milligram	mg	1/1,000 g	
Microgram	μg	10^{-6} g, 10^{-3} mg	
Nanogram	ng	10^{-9} g	
Picogram	pg	10^{-12} g	
Volume			
Liter	l		1.057 liquid qt
Deciliter	dl	1/100 l	
Milliliter	ml	1/1,000 l	
Microliter	μl	10^{-6} l, 10^{-3} ml	

*Extremely small figures are usually written as "$10^{-exponent}$." The number in the negative exponent indicates the number of digits to the right of the decimal point. For example, 10^{-6} m = 0.000,001 m (or 1/1,000,000 m). You may also see an expression such as 3×10^{-6}; this is equal to 0.000,003. Very large figures, on the other hand, are expressed by nonnegative exponents; in this case, the exponent indicates the number of digits to the right of the decimal. For instance, 3×10^6 = 300,000.0.

Weight Per Volume

One of the most frequently used measurements is weight per volume. Glucose, for example, is reported as milligrams per deciliter of whole blood or serum (mg/dl). (In older terminology, the results would be expressed as mg %.)

Volume Per Volume

Tests involving gases may be reported as volume of gas per volume of blood (or plasma or serum). For example, in the carbon dioxide—combining-power test, the results are expressed as the volume of carbon dioxide with which 1 dl blood serum or plasma will combine. A shorthand notation is vol %.

Partial Pressure

Another means of expressing the concentration of gases is in terms of partial pressure. Gases exert pressure because of the kinetic energy of the atoms or molecules of gas. In mixtures of gases, the pressure exerted by any one gas is expressed in relation to the amount present in the mixture. This quantity is called the partial pressure of the gas. Partial pressure is represented by the letter P with a subscript indicating the chemical symbol of the gas. For example, the partial pressure of carbon dioxide is symbolized as P_{CO_2}. Analyses of blood gases are reported in these terms.

Units Per Volume

Tests involving enzymes and some biologically active compounds and tests that give less precise measurements than can be determined by other means are reported as units per volume. In the case of enzyme-activity reports, this method is a shorthand notation; e.g., in the amylase test the units refer to the amount of starch reduced to glucose by the enzyme. Biologically active compounds such as follicle-stimulating hormone may be reported in international units (IU), based on standardized amounts required to elicit the appropriate response in the mouse ovary.

Milliequivalents Per Liter

To understand reports of electrolytes, one must understand the term "equivalent weight." It will be recalled from the study of chemistry that there are precise relationships between the amounts of elements or compounds that will react with one another. These amounts are determined by their atomic weights and their ability to combine (by gaining or losing electrons). Since the atomic weight of hydrogen is 1.008 and since it participates in many reactions, this element is used as the point of reference in determining equivalent weights. Thus, the weight in grams of an element or compound that will liberate or combine with one gram atomic weight of hydrogen, or hydrogen ion, is the gram equivalent weight of that substance. To illustrate this point, the following examples are given:

Combination of elements:

$H + Cl \rightarrow HCl$ — 1 g H combines with 35 g Cl; equivalent weight of Cl is 35.

$2H + O \rightarrow H_2O$ — 2 g H combines with 16 g O; equivalent weight of O is 8.

Liberation of hydrogen:

$Be + 2HCl \rightarrow BeCl_2 + H_2$ — 9.0 g Be liberates 2 g H; equivalent weight of Be is 4.5.

$Na + HCl \rightarrow NaCl + H$ — 23 g Na liberates 1 g H; equivalent weight of Na is 23.

Reaction of two compounds:

$NaOH + HCl \rightarrow NaCl + H_2O$ — One ion of Na replaces one ion of H; since one H ion is replaced, the equivalent weight of NaOH is the same as its molecular weight: 40.

$$2NaOH + H_2SO_4 \rightarrow Na_2SO_4 + 2H_2O$$

Two ions of Na replace two ions of H; since two ions of H are replaced, the equivalent weight of H_2SO_4 is one-half its molecular weight: 49.

The equivalent weight of an element of compound may also be determined by using valence. *Valence* is an expression of electric charge, indicated by the ability of elements or ions to gain or lose electrons. Thus, lithium, which loses only one electron, has a valence of 1. Calcium, on the other hand, loses two electrons and has a valence of 2. The equivalent weight is determined by dividing the atomic weight by the valence. Thus, the equivalent weight of lithium is $7 \div 1$, or 7; that of calcium is $40 \div 2$, or 20.

It must be remembered, however, that equivalent weights are influenced by the reactions in which the elements or compounds participate. This is illustrated by comparing two reactions in which ammonia participates. The decomposition of ammonia yields three hydrogen ions, making the equivalent weight of ammonia with respect to this reaction one-third the molecular weight: $17 \div 3$, or 5.67. However, when ammonia neutralizes hydrochloric acid, the equivalent weight is the same as the molecular weight because the reaction involves only one hydrogen ion.

The cardinal principle to remember about equivalents is that equal weights do not represent equal capacities for reaction. Not only is this evident in chemical reactions, but it is also seen in the effects on osmotic pressure (both these effects are extremely important in physiologic considerations). Consideration of osmotic-pressure changes shows, for instance, that sulfuric acid, which yields three ions on ionization, has more effect on osmotic pressure than does hydrochloric acid, which yields but two ions.

From the consideration of equivalents and osmotic-pressure effects, it is apparent that weight-per-weight or weight-per-volume expressions of concentrations do not describe these functions adequately. To use an everyday analogy, one invites an equal number of boys and girls to a dance; one would not arrange for 1,400 lb of boys and 1,400 lb of girls and expect an equal number of each to be present.

The magnitude of concentrations of electrolytes in the human body is such that it is easier to express them as milliequivalents (meq) rather than as equivalents. A similar relation in magnitude is shown by comparing milligrams with grams. The electrolytes considered here include sodium, potassium, calcium, chloride, and phosphate.

Number Per Volume

Especially important in hematology is the quantitative measure of number per volume. For example, counts of blood cells are reported as number of cells per cubic millimeter of whole blood. In urinalysis, reports of the microscopic examination of sediment (formed elements) are expressed as number per high- or low-power field of the microscope, and a range is indicated when there are less than 50 percent, such as 2 to 4 WBC/hpf (white blood cells per high-power field). When innumerable particular formed elements are present, it is common to indicate this by the notation "full field." The use of range is a means to indicate the variation that may be noted in scanning the number of fields in order to have reasonable assessment of the sediment. White and red cell estimations are reported per high-power field; casts and epithelial cells per low-power field.

The relative term "percent" is used in reporting results of study of stained blood smears. A minimum of 100 white blood cells is counted, keeping a tabulation of the number of each of the various types of cells seen. Since the basic number counted is 100, the numbers of individual types are the percent figures. When nucleated red blood cells are present, they are reported as the number seen while counting 100 white blood cells.

Rank Order

Rough approximations are often stated in rank-order units or as qualifying adjectives. Rank-order units used are the following:

trace, 1+, 2+, 3+, and 4+; the higher the number, the greater the amount present. Qualifying adjectives include slight, moderate, and marked. These terms are used to indicate the degree of abnormality, e.g., moderate hypochromasia of red blood cells.

Titer

This term is used particularly in serologic test reports. It is defined as the last dilution at which a reaction takes place, i.e., the end point of the reaction. For example, agglutination tests are reported as a ratio between serum and diluent. Thus, a serum which has been diluted 1 part in 256 parts diluent and still demonstrates agglutination of the test antigen would be reported as positive 1:256.

NORMAL RANGE

All laboratory tests have, as a prerequisite to their proper interpretation, normal ranges. A range is necessary because of individual differences even among a normal population. In addition, there is no test which can be said to be so accurate that an absolute value is possible. The normal range establishes the area within which one may be confident in saying that no pathologic condition exists.

The normal range must be determined for two purposes: discrimination and description. By discrimination, we mean that it separates the normal from the truly abnormal. By description, we mean that it tells us what we can expect of the normal population. The narrower the range, the more discriminating it is. For example, the normal range for blood glucose by the Somogyi method is 65 to 100 mg/dl blood; that for urea nitrogen is 8 to 28 mg/dl blood. An example of descriptive data is seen in blood grouping. There is no true normal range in the usual sense, but only in the incidence of certain major blood groups within a given ethnic population. For example, group B is more common among Oriental than among Caucasian populations.

With the advent of automation, it has become possible to screen large numbers of individuals and, in the process, establish the base line for those individuals. This is an important contribution to improvement of health care because it allows the physician to compare the individual with his *own* normal range. For example, the normal base-line value for a given individual's lactic acid dehydrogenase may be at the extreme low point of the normal range for the general population. Thus he could develop an elevation due to a disease process that is significant and still be within the normal range of the general population.

Determination of Normal Range

To establish a normal range, a large enough sample of normal individuals must be tested; then the data must be analyzed statistically to interpret the distribution of values obtained. A simple method is to tabulate values in rank order from highest to lowest and set the normal limits between the 95th and 5th percentiles. Any value above the 95th percentile would be considered out of normal range, and, similarly, any value below the 5th percentile would also be considered abnormal. Gaussian distribution—the so-called "normal curve"—is also useful in determining normal range. In plotting the distribution of frequency of occurrence of any measure in graphic form, a bell-shaped curve, as shown in Fig. 1-1, is characteristic of normal distribution. The highest point of the curve is the mean. Points on either side of this are plotted from calculations of the standard deviation for a given set of data on a given test. Standard deviation is an expression of the variation around a measure of central tendency, the mean.

In the laboratory, the principle of the standard deviation (σ) is used to determine normal range and to monitor performance. The usual limits for normal range are 2.5 σ above, and 2.5 σ below the mean. This has been chosen largely on the basis of probability. At ± 1 σ, one-third of the values will be outside the limits, and thus the range within the limits is not an accurate description of the normal population. At ± 2 σ, 20 percent of the values will be outside the limits; although ± 2 σ produces a more descriptive normal range, the values outside of the range are still too large. At ± 2.5 σ, only 0.5 percent of the values are outside the limits, and thus a reasonable and accurate description of normal range is

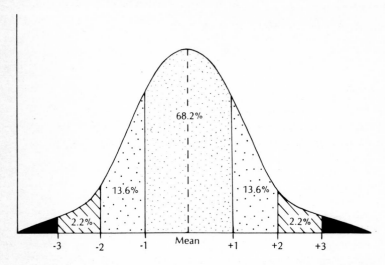

FIG. 1-1 Normal bell curve.

obtained. At ±3 σ, there is 0.15 percent chance of random error causing a value to be beyond the limits. While it eliminates the possibility of being outside the range without overt error, it may give too wide a range, even beyond biologically determined normals, leading to the chance of not detecting an abnormal value. The principle of standard deviation is applicable to detection of error in the test system and depends on the maintenance of detailed records to diagnose and correct aberration.

Allowable Limits of Error

Another approach to defining the limits within which error may be tolerated is by determining the allowable limits of error in a procedure. This calculation involves the *mean* and the *range* of the normal biologic range. For example, if the normal biologic range is 80 to 100 mg/dl, the *range* is 20 (obtained by subtracting the lower limit from the upper limit). The *mean* is (80 + 100) ÷ 2, a value of 90. The equation for calculating the allowable limits of error in percent is:

$$X = \frac{B/4}{x_n} \times 100$$

X = allowable limits in %

B = range

x_n = mean

Example

A sample is tested for glucose and found to have a value of 88 mg/dl. The known concentration of this sample is 95 mg/dl. The normal range for glucose according to the method used is 60 to 100 mg/dl.

$$B = 100 - 60 = 40$$

$$x_n = \frac{100 + 60}{2} = 80$$

Substituting the known values in the above equiation and solving for X:

$$X = \frac{40/4}{80} \times 100 = \frac{10}{80} \times 100 = 12\%$$

Since this is the allowable limit in percent, the next step is to find the mg/dl which this represents. The value of the known concentration is multiplied by 0.12, and the result 10.4 mg/dl, is used to define the limits.

```
 95.0      95.0
-10.4      10.4
-----     -----
 84.6     105.4
```

The allowable limits of error in milligrams per deciliter, then, are from 84.6 to 105.4. With this information, we find that the result of 88 mg/dl, while not the true value, is within the allowable limits of error. Some laboratories include this type of information on the report forms as an aid to the physician in interpreting serial determinations on a single patient.

QUALITY CONTROL

Quality control involves the application of all means possible to guarantee that the results reported by the laboratory are both reliable and valid. Reliability concerns the consistency of the work; a component of reliability is precision, which is the degree to which a result can be reproduced using the same sample. Validity concerns the degree to which the test measures what it is supposed to measure with accuracy. Accuracy is the degree to which the test results approximates the "true" (absolute) value. Elements that contribute to quality control include:

1. Personal attitude of the worker. If he assumes that he "knows it all," there is no room for improvement because he will not admit to its possibility and is unwilling to be checked.
2. Procedure. Accuracy depends on the technologist's thorough knowledge of technical aspects, skill in performance, and sound judgment.
3. Equipment. It is false security to assume that one standardization or calibration of an instrument lasts throughout its life.
4. Standards. The mere labeling of a standard solution does not give it the magic quality of infallibility. Shelf life is not interminable.
5. Reagents. All materials used in performing tests must be accurately prepared. Shelf life, again, is critical. In all laboratory procedures, the reactants in reagents must be checked with known samples to make sure they are giving true reactions. For example, in bacteriology, false negative results because of error in the culture medium could lead to invalid or missed identification of organisms.
6. Calculations. Arithmetical error is one of the common sources of error.

Preparation and Collection

One of the most important factors in the accuracy of laboratory and radiologic tests is the proper preparation of the patient and collection of specimens. Information about the patient's diagnosis and treatment regimen can also be extremely useful. For example, consider the following situation: The physician requests that an electrolyte-determination test be done on a patient who is receiving intravenous fluids containing electrolytes. It would be worse than useless to obtain the blood specimen from the needle through which the infusion is being administered. The specimen would be contaminated by the solution, rendering false high results. It is permissible to draw the sample from the opposite arm, but the requisition and report should include a notation concerning the fact that an infusion was in process. Otherwise, the physician could be misled by the results, since the true physiologic condition of the patient is not represented under such circumstances.

The laboratory may request collection of another sample or prepare the patient again for a procedure if the first sample is not satisfactory. The reason(s) for the sample's not being satisfactory should be explained so that errors will not be repeated. An example of improper processing of a specimen is to be seen in the blood urea nitrogen test. The test involves the nitrogen fraction of the urea molecule. Thus if whole blood rather than serum is to be used, the choice of anticoagulant is critical. If an ammonium oxalate is used for the anticoagulant, false high results will be obtained, since ammonium contains nitrogen.

Influence of Drugs

There are a number of problems in quality control which demand greater communication with, and use of the expertise of, the pharmacist. It has long been recognized that drugs the patient may be taking can influence the results of tests to the point of yielding misleading information. As often as possible, such influences are noted in the procedure protocol and instructions for preparation of patients. One cannot assume, however, that all the possibilities have been covered, for the development of new drugs and the use of drugs in combination, for individual patient needs, can easily make these notations obsolete.

The clinician's interpretation of results can be sharpened, and the pathologist and medical technologist can extend the comprehensiveness of their evaluation of results that are "out of control" due to drug interference, if a pharmacist can take an active part in solving problems. The need for vigilance and good communication point up the common saying that, as specialization increases, so does interdependence. Pooling of knowledge and expertise provides more effective functioning and better patient care.

SIGNIFICANCE OF CHANGES IN SERIAL DETERMINATIONS

In monitoring treatment or progress of the patient, an indicator test (or tests) may be used, e.g., hemoglobin in anemia. Accuracy and precision are the foundation of the validity of such judgments. These two qualities of a test procedure must, of course, be as near the ideal, as possible. There is no procedure which does not have some sources of error. Keeping these at a reasonable and identifiable level is the responsibility of the laboratory. Assuming this, the interpretation of the significance of change in a patient must be made with the understanding that some of the variation can be due to inherent error. By no means is all variation accounted for in this way. Other variations must be attributable to a change in the patient.

As an example of the interpretation of changes, let us consider hemoglobin. In the past, when the methods for this test were relatively (if not absolutely!) crude, hematologists considered a change of ±1 g/dl necessary before change could be considered significant. With better instruments and more precision, a change of ±0.3 g/dl can be considered significant, i.e., a true change in the patient rather than an error inherent in the method.

SCREENING TESTS

The purpose of screening tests, no matter what the type, is to identify actual or potential disease states in large, apparently healthy populations. The routine periodic physical examination may be considered such a procedure, and it frequently involves laboratory and radiologic examinations. Although health care nowadays emphasizes therapy, there is a gradual shift toward preventive medicine. This is seen in several ways, such as inoculations against infectious diseases, nutrition education, and identification of conditions predisposing to disease. The latter problem is particularly susceptible to solution by use of screening tests. As the means to conduct numerous tests on relatively small amounts of specimen and at reasonable costs are becoming available, screening tests are being used with increasing frequency.

The accuracy of a screening test depends on its specificity and sensitivity. Freeman and Beeler[1] define diagnostic *specificity* of tests as "the ability of the test to yield a negative result for patients without the disease" and express the definition quantitatively as

$$100\% = \frac{\text{no. of positive test results in patients without the disease}}{\text{no. of people tested without the disease}} \times 100$$

If the test is 100 percent specific, there will be no false positives. *Sensitivity,* on the other hand, is the degree to which the test detects disease without yielding false negatives. It is expressed quantitatively as

$$100\% = \frac{\text{no. of negative test results in patients with the disease}}{\text{no. of people tested with the disease}} \times 100$$

The test is 100 percent sensitive if no false negatives are obtained.

Freeman and Beeler define diagnostic *accuracy* as "the ability of the test to classify the entire population tested for the disease in question." They note that, because most diseases have a relatively low incidence among the total population, "accuracy depends more on specificity than on sensitivity."

[1] J. A. Freeman and M. F. Beeler, "Laboratory Medicine—Clinical Microscopy," p. 175, Lea & Febiger, Philadelphia, 1974.

Obviously, the establishment, by these definitions, of the diagnostic sensitivity and accuracy of the many screening tests available depends on amassing a great deal of data from many subjects. Those tests that have been validated by statistical data are so designated in the instructions that come with the test kit. Tests that have not yet been so validated can be used in diagnosis, but the interpretation of the results is subject to the clinician's judgment.

TWO

URINE EXAMINATIONS

Lowly though its status may be in the eyes of some, urine is one of the most remarkable and important fluids of the body. The need to maintain the delicate balance of water and electrolytes, and to rid the body of waste products as well as toxic elements makes the excretion of urine essential to the economy of the body. As shown in Table 2-1, the formation of urine is, of itself, a remarkable process involving filtration and secretion and reabsorption of essential components. These processes are governed by the hydrostatic and osmotic pressure of the renal blood supply and by the secretion of hormones. Thus urine is a valuable and abundant source of information about many biologic processes seemingly unrelated to kidney function. Its importance has been recognized since ancient times, increasing with the sophistication of instruments and knowledge of physiology and pathophysiology.

TABLE 2-1   THE FORMATION OF URINE

Anatomical area	Event
Bowman's capsule	Formation of plasma ultrafiltrate, at an average rate of 130 ml/min
Proximal convo-luted tubules	1. Reabsorption of "threshold" substances (glucose, creatine, amino acids, vitamin C, lactate, pyruvate) by tubular cells by means of enzymatic transport systems 2. Active secretion of some substances by tubular cells and/or excretion of materials derived from peritubu-lar interstitial fluid 3. Reabsorption of at least 85% of the water and of some sodium chloride and other electrolytes. This reabsorption is obligatory, i.e., not governed by the body's need for water and electrolytes.
Loop of Henle	Further reabsorption of water by the mechanism of countercurrent exchanges. By this stage, 90% of the water has been reabsorbed, and the original volume has been reduced to 13–16 ml/min
Distal convoluted tubule	Facultative absorption of water and electrolytes, gov-erned by the body's needs as reflected in the stimula-tion of the posterior pituitary to release antidiuretic hormone
Collecting tubule	Completion of the transformation of the filtrate to urine. The volume is now 1 ml/min, and the concen-tration of excretory substances is greatly increased.

COLLECTION OF SPECIMEN

No test is any more accurate than the way in which the speci-men submitted for analysis is collected. In urinalysis, time is a critical factor with respect to when the specimen is collected and when the analysis is begun. Urine deteriorates relatively rapidly; therefore, single specimens (i.e., not timed or long-period speci-mens) should be analyzed as soon after collection as possible. The manner in which the urine specimen is collected is of critical importance to certain types of analysis. Careful attention must be paid to these details if the information obtained from the tests is to be accurate enough to allow the making of sound diagnos-tic and therapeutic decisions. One of four major types of specimen may be required:

Single, random specimens, no special preparation required
Timed, short-period specimens
Timed, long-period specimens
Specimens for microbiological examinations

The container used to collect and/or deliver the specimen to the laboratory is of primary concern. Clean, wide-mouthed containers of adequate size are a must for collection, although smaller containers that are specifically designed for urine samples may be used for the portion submitted for analysis.

Random Specimens

Since the composition of urine is subject to diet and water intake and therefore varies during a given period, the time of collection of random samples influences the results. First, the relation of time to physiologic processes influences what may be expected in terms of pathologic amounts of constituents (normal or abnormal). For example, the first morning sample is useful because it is most likely to be most concentrated, have an acid pH, and contain formed elements associated with infection. It is less likely to reveal threshhold substances related to diet and metabolism such as glucose. When the urine is dilute (i.e., specific gravity of less than 1.010), small but significant pathologic amounts of constituents may not be detectable. At alkaline pH, which is common after meals, important formed elements such as casts may be destroyed. These considerations must be taken into account, and the patient must be instructed to collect the specimen which is optimal in revealing the presence of pathologic or diagnostic elements. When such care is taken, the absence of such elements can more safely be interpreted as ruling out or confirm the absence of disease.

Timed, Short-period Specimens

Directions for specimen collections for short periods (usually 2 h) are provided in the discussions of tests involving this type of specimen, since there are variations related to the constituent sought.

Timed, Long-period Specimens

Depending on the type of analysis to be performed, 12- or 24-h urine specimens require some manner of preservation to inhibit bacterial growth and/or maintain the constituent(s) sought. Refrigeration, in combination with the appropriate additive, is a common procedure. The laboratory will provide the large specimen bottle(s), the appropriate preservative, and directions, including specifications on water intake, to be given to the patient. It is essential that the patient understand that *all the urine voided* in the specified period is saved because tests with time-period specimens are reported in terms of total output in the period and thus depend on the laboratory's having the total volume voided. Otherwise, erroneous values could be reported, and interpretation of results could cause a possible error in diagnosis.

1. General instructions
   - *a.* Give the patient a bottle large enough to accommodate the entire specimen.
   - *b.* Keep the specimen cold during the collection period.
   - *c.* Caution the patient to collect urine before defecating.
   - *d.* Use preservatives according to laboratory instructions.
2. Method of collection
   - *a.* Have the patient void at the beginning of the test period (usually at 7 or 8 A.M.); then discard the specimen.
   - *b.* For 24-h specimens, collect all urine voided between the beginning of the test period and the same hour the following day, pouring each voiding into the large bottle provided.
   - *c.* End the collection period by having the patient collect the last voiding at the same hour the day following the beginning of the collection period.

Collection of Specimens for Cultures

ROUTINE BACTERIOLOGIC CULTURES

Collection of urine specimens for culture requires the utmost cooperation of the nurse, since it is almost invariably she or he who instructs the patient and gives him the equipment. The nurse must keep in mind that it is one of the procedures in which contamination of the specimen can most easily, though inadvertently, happen. Special care must be taken when handling the bottle and cap to maintain sterility. The specimen should be taken to the laboratory immediately, so that the culture may be started before contaminating organisms that might have been introduced have time to grow sufficiently to produce erroneous results.

In women, catheterization was once considered essential in order to avoid contamination of the specimen, especially from vaginal secretions, and because it is difficult to clean the area surrounding the urethral orifice. However, nowadays the trend is toward the simpler procedure of a clean-voided midstream specimen, as it has been found that contamination of the bladder may result from catheterization. Obviously, it is less objectionable to contaminate the specimen than the bladder.

The specimens are collected as follows:

1. Female
   a. Clean the entire vulvar area, using soap and water followed by Zephiran Chloride.
   b. With the labia held apart, have the patient void directly into the sterile bottle after passing some urine, collecting the midstream portion of the voiding.
   c. Cap the bottle with a sterile cap and take it directly to the laboratory.
   d. Note the method of collection of all specimens for culture.
2. Male
   a. Clean the meatus and surrounding parts well with soap and water followed by Zephiran Chloride.
   b. Have the patient void directly into a sterile bottle after passing some urine, collecting the midstream portion of the voiding.

CULTURES FOR TUBERCLE BACILLI

For cultures for tubercle bacilli, a first morning specimen (preferably catheterized) is now recommended in preference to the previously used 24-h specimen. It has been found that urine itself is toxic to tubercle bacilli, and therefore the 24-h specimen may give misleading results, since many bacilli die during the period of collection before they can be cultured. Catheterization is necessary in order to eliminate contamination with acid-fast saprophytes.

PHYSIOLOGIC CONSTITUENTS OF URINE

The physiologic constituents of urine include organic and inorganic compounds, and those present in the greatest amounts are water (90 to 95 percent), urea, uric acid, creatinine, chloride, sodium, potassium, phosphates, and ammonia. Normally only traces of a number of other compounds are present. Under pathologic conditions, urine includes other substances related to specific disease processes and/or abnormally high amounts of a normal constituent. An example of the former is protein, as in the proteinuria associated with nephritis; an example of the latter is calcium, which is excreted in large amounts in hyperparathyroid conditions. Since the composition and volume of urine are influenced by fluid intake, diet, etc., normal values for the various constituents are expressed as the average and are determined from the 24-h output (Table 2-2).

TABLE 2-2
COMPOSITION OF A TYPICAL NORMAL URINE (DAILY EXCRETION)

Substance	Amount, g	Substance	Amount, g
Water	1,200.0	Chloride (as NaCl)	12.0
Solids	60.0	Sodium	4.0
Urea	30.0	Phosphate (as P)	1.1
Uric acid	0.7	Potassium	2.0
Hippuric acid	0.27	Calcium	0.2
Creatinine	1.2	Magnesium	0.15
Indican	0.01	Sulfur (as S)	1.0
Oxalic acid	0.02	Inorganic sulfur	0.8
Allantoin	0.04	Neutral sulfur	0.12
Amino acid nitrogen	0.2	Conjugated sulfates	0.08
Purine bases	0.01	Ammonia	0.7
Phenols	0.2		

SOURCE: After B. L. Oser (ed.), "Hawk's Practical Physiological Chemistry," 14th ed., © 1965 by McGraw-Hill, Inc. Used with permission of McGraw-Hill Book Company.

ROUTINE URINALYSIS

The patient is given a clean, wide-mouthed bottle and is instructed to void directly into it. If he is to collect the specimen at home, he should be requested to use a small clean jar and bring the specimen to the laboratory as soon as possible. Patients have been known to use perfume bottles and other such containers, which are difficult to empty and which may be contaminated by the original contents, rendering the specimen unsatisfactory for examination.

The usual tests in routine urinalysis include a description of its color and degree of cloudiness (if any), the pH (acidity or alkalinity), specific gravity, tests for protein, test for glucose, and a microscopic examination of the sediment. The findings of these routine tests may indicate the need for other tests.

Appearance

The color of the specimen may range from pale straw (dilute specimen) to dark amber (concentrated specimen); under the influence of various drugs, foods, and diseases, the color may be quite different from the normal straw color. Table 2-3 gives a correlation of urine color with specific conditions. Cloudiness of a urine specimen may be due to precipitated crystals such as amorphous phosphates or urates, or to many epithelial, pus, or red blood cells, or to bacteria.

Acidity or Alkalinity (pH)

Normal range: 4.5–7.5

The expression pH is a measure of the hydrogen-ion concentration and indicates the degree of acidity or alkalinity of a solution. The complete range of pH values is from 1 to 14. The lower the number, the greater the acidity (i.e., hydrogen-ion concentration). In urinalysis, pH determination may be done roughly or exactly. In a rough determination litmus paper is used as the indicator, showing whether the specimen is acid or alkaline. The test results with litmus paper are simply reported as "acid" or "alkaline." An

TABLE 2-3   COLOR OF URINE IN VARIOUS CONDITIONS

Color	Cause of coloration	Pathologic condition
Nearly colorless	Dilution or diminution of normal pigments	Nervous conditions, hydruria, diabetes insipidus, granular kidney
Dark yellow to amber	Increase of normal, or occurrence of pathologic, pigments; concentrated urine	Acute febrile diseases
Milky	Fat globules, pus cells, amorphous phosphate	Chyluria, purulent diseases of the urinary tract
Orange	Excreted drugs, such as santonin, chrysophanic acid, pyridine	
Red or reddish	Hematoporphyrin, hemoglobin, myoglobin, erythrocytes	Hemorrhage, hemoglobinuria, trauma
Brown to brown-black	Hematin, methemoglobin, melanin, hydroquinone, pyrocatechol	Hemorrhage, methemoglobinuria, melanotic sarcoma
Greenish-yellow or brown, approaching black	Bile pigments	Phenol poisoning, jaundice
Dirty green or blue (dark-blue surface scum, blue deposit)	Excess of indigo-forming substances, methylene blue medication	Cholera; typhus (seen especially when urine is putrefying)

SOURCE: From B. L. Oser (ed.), "Hawk's Practical Physiological Chemistry," 14th ed., © 1965 by McGraw-Hill, Inc. Used with permission of McGraw-Hill Book Company.

exact pH determination may be made with a special indicator, Nitrazine, which shows a series of colors (yellow, green, and blue) corresponding to pH values. The Combistix[1] reagent strip uses a combination of methyl red and bromthymol blue in the determination of pH. This combination of dyes gives a series of colors (bright orange, yellow, green, and blue) within the range of pH

[1] Combistix is the product of the Ames Company, Elkhart, Ind.

TABLE 2-4 CONDITIONS CONDUCIVE TO CONSISTENT pH

pH	Condition
Above 6.0	1. Certain bacterial infections of the urinary system (e.g., Bacillus proteus)
	2. Alkalosis
	a. Hyperventilation
	b. Hyperemesis
	c. Large doses of alkali (e.g., sodium bicarbonate)
	d. Excessive ingestion of potassium salts
	3. Potassium depletion
	a. Renal insufficiency
	b. Hyperaldosteronism
	c. Prolonged therapy with cortisone or carbonic anhydrase inhibitors
Below 6.0	1. Metabolic acidosis
	2. Respiratory acidosis
	3. Pyrexia
	4. Metabolic disorders
	a. Phenylketonuria
	b. Alkaptonuria
	5. Methyl alcohol poisoning

SOURCE: After R. M. Kark et al., "A Primer of Urinalysis," 2d ed., Harper & Row, Publishers, Incorporated, Hoeber Medical Division, New York, 1963.

4 to 9. Normal urine has a pH between 6 and 7. A pH value of less than 6.0 is considered acid, and a value above 7.0 is considered alkaline.

Information about pH is essential to the evaluation of microscopic examinations of the urine. The pH determines whether certain formed elements are preserved or destroyed and aids in the identification of crystals. Casts and the cellular elements of the urinary sediment are preserved in an acid pH, but they readily disintegrate in alkaline pH.

There are certain clinical indications for maintaining the patient's urinary pH at either acid or alkaline levels. For example, in the treatment of hypertension with mecamylamine, control is most effective and fewer side effects develop if the patient's urine is maintained without fluctuation of pH. The drug is excreted when the urine is acid and tends to be retained when it is alkaline. Table 2-5

TABLE 2-5   CONDITIONS REQUIRING CONTROL OF
URINARY pH IN THERAPY

Optimal pH	Condition
Above 6.0	1. Management of calculi formed in acid urines
	2. Streptomycin therapy of urinary system. (The drug is effective only in alkaline urine.)
	3. Sulfonamide therapy. (Alkaline pH prevents precipitation of crystals of the drug in the urinary tract.)
	4. Treatment of salicylate intoxication
	5. Treatment of blood-transfusion reactions. (Alkaline urine is considered protective against renal damage.)
	6. Treatment of hypertension with mecamylamine (see text)
Below 6.0	1. Management of calculi formed in alkaline urines
	2. Treatment of urinary-tract infections due to urea-splitting organisms (e.g., Bacillus proteus)

SOURCE: After R. M. Kark et al., "A Primer of Urinalysis," 2d ed., Harper & Row, Publishers, Incorporated, Hoeber Medical Division, New York, 1963.

shows the principal conditions in which regulation of pH is an important part of therapy. Urinary pH may be maintained at alkaline levels by a diet emphasizing citrus fruits and most vegetables while reducing intake of acid-producing foods. Alkali salts, such as potassium citrate, are prescribed. Acid levels may be maintained by a diet rich in proteins and poor in foods resulting in alkaline output. Ammonium chloride, ammonium nitrate, and sodium acid phosphate are drugs used to enhance an acid pH.

Specific Gravity

Normal range: 1.010–1.025

When substances are dissolved in a liquid, the weight of the solution thus formed is increased proportionately. *Specific gravity* is the term used to indicate the degree of concentration of a solution. Water is used as the basis of comparison, distilled water having a specific gravity of 1.000 g/ml. In other words, 1 ml water weighs 1 g.

Specific gravity is measured by the hydrometer, an instrument which contains a mercury bulb attached to a stem with a graduated scale indicating a range of concentration from 1.000 to 1.040. When used to measure specific gravity of urine, the hydrometer is commonly called a urinometer (see Fig. 2-1). The principle by which this instrument functions is displacement; i.e., the more concentrated the solution, the more the instrument floating in the solution is displaced upward. This is a rather crude measurement, but its simplicity has made it a useful tool. One disadvantage of this method is that it requires a minimum of 20 ml of specimen. Whenever there is less than this amount of specimen, it is noted on the report as qns. − quantity not sufficient.

Measurement of the concentration of solutions may be made by more precise means than the hydrometer. In addition to being more precise, these methods do not require relatively large amounts of specimen, an obvious advantage, particularly in pediatric cases. The methods which are coming into more common use are the refractive index and osmolality.

REFRACTIVE INDEX

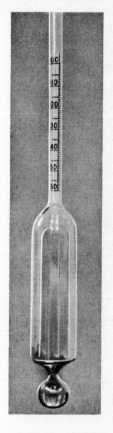

FIG. 2-1 The urinometer. (Courtesy of *The Clinical Laboratory*, St. Louis.)

Light waves are bent (refracted) as they pass obliquely from one medium to another of different density, in which their speed is different, or through layers of different density in the same medium. A common illustration of this principle is the broken appearance of a pencil placed in water—the portion not underwater appears to be displaced to the side of the portion underwater. Differences in density between air and water account for this refraction.

The instrument used in determining the concentration of urine samples by this principle is the refractometer. This instrument has a light source which passes through a chamber containing the specimen and a prism with a scale indicating the degree of refraction of the light as it emerges from the specimen. There is a direct relationship between this reading and the concentration of the sample. Thus, the readings of the refractometer can be converted into specific gravity. This is a precise measure and requires only a drop of sample—both important advantages in urinalysis.

OSMOLALITY

Osmolality, by definition, is a functional relationship between the number of particles[1] present in a solution and the effect of these particles on the colligative properties of the solution. Solutions have definite and measurable colligative properties: vapor pressure, osmotic pressure, boiling point, and freezing point. These are determined routinely in many types of analysis. For example, the more particles present in a solution, no matter what their size, the greater the depression of the freezing point. Measurement of the freezing point thus affords a precise means of determining concentration of solutions, of which urine is an example.

By definition, one osmol equals ϕn moles, where ϕ is the osmotic coefficient, and n is the number of ions into which a molecule dissociates in solution. Since 1 mol of a nonionic solute will depress the freezing point of 1 kg of water 1.86°C, 1 *osmol* of *any* solute will lower the freezing point by this amount. A milliosmol (mOsm) is 1/1,000 of an osmol. In biologic samples, the degree of magnitude is in terms of milliosmols, and this is the unit of measure reported. For comparison of the milliosmol with the more familiar specific gravity, 290 mOsm/liter is equivalent to a specific gravity of about 1.010.

USEFULNESS OF SPECIFIC GRAVITY

The specific gravity of urine varies throughout the day according to the concentration, determined in large measure by the fluid

---

[1] Particles here refer to molecules (e.g., glucose) and/or ions (e.g., Na^+ or Cl^-).

intake. The mechanism of concentration and dilution of the urine is related to the activity of the tubular epithelium in excretion or reabsorption of water. The glomerular filtrate has a specific gravity of about 1.010. As the fluid progresses along the renal system, water is reabsorbed or excreted under the influence of the body's needs. With reabsorption, the urine becomes more concentrated, and thus the specific gravity becomes higher. If the need is to rid the body of fluid, the urine is diluted, bringing the specific gravity to lower values.

A test for specific gravity may serve several functions. First, it is important to have information on the specific gravity of the specimen when evaluating microscopic examinations of the sediment. In extremely dilute specimens (1.005 or lower), some of the elements, particularly red cells and casts, will be ruptured, and a false negative results will be obtained. Second, tests of the specific gravity of urine reveal the ability of the kidneys to concentrate or dilute the urine, according to the needs of the body. When the ability to concentrate urine is impaired, active renal disease should be suspected. To illustrate the importance of this simple test, the following case history is cited:

History

A 19-year-old female, 4½-months pregnant, presented to the University Hospital with a history of being well until 4 days previously, when she experienced right-lower-abdominal and right-flank pain in association with severe frontal headaches, chills, fever, vomiting, anorexia, and diarrhea. She stated that she had voided an adequate amount of urine throughout the course of this illness.

Physical Examination

Revealed a temperature of 103.4°F., a pulse of 110 per minute, a blood pressure of 90/50, a uterus enlarged to 4½-months pregnant, severe right-lower-quadrant and right-flank pain, and clinical evidence of marked dehydration. Catheterization of the urinary bladder yielded approximately 25 ml of cloudy urine that showed 30 to 40 WBC/hpf, with clumps of WBC and large, coarsely granular casts, pus casts, and bacilli. A blood urea nitrogen (BUN) performed at this time was reported as 40 mg/dl.

Hospital Course

A diagnosis of pyelonephritis of pregnancy in association with severe dehydration was made, and replacement-fluid therapy and antibiotics begun. In spite of fluid administration, the urine output remained fixed at 5 to 10 ml/h for the next several hours, and a specific gravity of 1.007 was reported. This low specific gravity in the presence of dehydration and oliguria pointed to acute renal failure. The program of therapy was immediately changed from one of rehydration to one of judicious fluid administration, as befits the conditions of acute renal shutdown. During the next several days, the patient was closely followed with hourly urine measurements, daily BUNs, and daily urine specific gravities, represented in the table below.

Hospital day	Urine specific gravity	BUN, ml/dl
1	1.013	41
2	1.007	51
3	1.006	63
4	1.004	—
5	1.004	70
6	1.003	65
7	1.009	45
8	1.013	49
14	1.014	20
15	1.015	16

Comment

The specific gravity of urine was the "open sesame" in this case. A poorly concentrated urine in the presence of clinical dehydration was the first clue to renal failure. How long would the diagnosis have been delayed if the specimen had been reported "quantity not sufficient"? This patient could have been given fluids in a vigorous effort to correct her clinical dehydration, until overloading and fatal pulmonary edema developed.[1]

Chemical Analysis

PROTEIN

Normal range
24-h specimen: none
Random sample:[2] male: none to slight trace
female: none to trace voided

Although most urinalysis reports list a test for albumin rather than a test for protein, it is better to refer to this as a protein test, since albumin is but one protein that may be found in the urine. Other proteins, such as globulin and fibrinogen, may also be found.

Most tests for protein are based upon the phenomenon of coagulation of the protein, either by heat or by chemical agents. The cloudiness thus produced is estimated qualitatively and expressed as trace, 1+, 2+, 3+, and 4+. For accurate quantitative determinations, specified amounts of specimen and reagents as well as precise measurement of the resulting precipitated protein are necessary.

In the Combistix[3] or Urostix[3] reagent-strip tests, the presence of protein is detected by a change in the color of an indicator. The principle of this test is found in the "protein error of indicators." At a fixed pH, certain indicators will have one color in the presence of protein and a different color in the absence of protein. The reagent strip contains a citrate buffer and bromphenol blue. The citrate buffer provides a pH of approximately 3.0, and at this

[1] Gilder L. Wideman, The Importance of "Simple" Laboratory Tests, *Alabama J. Med. Technol.*, 1(1):11, 1959.

[2] In a random sample, less specific reagents are usually employed for screening purposes, and compounds other than true protein can give these slight positive results; hence the apparent discrepancy between the normal results of random and 24-h samples.

[3] Combistix and Urostix are products of the Ames Company, Elkhart, Inc.

pH the indicator has a yellow color when no protein is present. With increasing amounts of protein, the color change is through green to blue.

This method of testing for proteinuria is more specific than the tests based on turbidity. In addition, it is not affected by cloudiness of the specimen or interfering substances. The reagent strips are stable when protected in their original container and kept under normal temperature and humidity.

In quantitative measurement of protein, a 24-h specimen is necessary. No preservative should be added to the specimen, and it must be kept cold in order to inhibit bacterial growth. The bottle used should be large enough to accommodate the entire 24-h output, so that mixture of the specimen is complete, permitting an accurate test result.

Protein enters the urine in several ways. For example, pressure on the renal blood supply can result in "leaking" of some of the plasma protein into the glomerular system, giving a positive test for protein in the urine. This case is not one of intrinsic renal disease. When there is damage to the renal system and a consequent breakdown of cellular integrity, plasma proteins are lost into the urine. This and bleeding into the urine are particularly indicative of nephritis. Sometimes the loss of plasma proteins in nephritis can be severe enough to cause hypoproteinemia. Proteinuria may be seen in glomerulosclerosis and results from renal anoxia associated with this condition.

Not all proteinuria has its origin in the kidneys, however. Inflammatory processes anywhere in the urinary system and its closely associated structures (such as the prostate and epididymis) can lead to proteinuria, because purulent secretions can produce proteinuria: there is injury to the inflamed cells, and the disintegrating pus and blood cells that are present contribute to the protein.

Periodic testing of the urine for protein is done, with other pertinent clinical tests, to detect any signs of impending toxemia during pregnancy. Proteinuria is a consistent finding in toxemia of pregnancy, and this testing is a valuable check on such a development.

Bence-Jones Protein

This compound was discovered by Henry Bence-Jones in 1848. It is associated with bone tumors (principally multiple myeloma) and may be present in hyperparathyroidism and osteomalacia. Its excretion in the urine is variable, and thus diagnosis of conditions in which it may be present in the urine is not dependent upon a positive result. The molecular weight of Bence-Jones protein is 34,000, making it much more easily excreted in the urine because of its relatively low molecular weight and size, as compared with albumin (70,000) and globulin (165,000). This protein has characteristic physical properties which aid in its detection. It is precipitated at temperatures between 45 and 70°C and disappears again at 100°C.

Electrophoretic Analysis

There may be times when it is valuable to know the relative amounts of different proteins present in the urine. This may be determined by electrophoretic separation (see Chap. 3 for a detailed discussion of electrophoresis).

GLUCOSE

Normal range: none

Ordinarily the presence of glucose in the urine indicates diabetes mellitus, but this is not invariably true. There are some cases in which the renal threshold, i.e., the blood glucose level at which glucose is spilled over into the urine, is low. Some persons may, therefore, have a positive reaction but no intrinsic disease. Thus, it is wise to check several specimens taken at different times of the day, as well as the blood glucose levels, in order to rule out the possibility of disease.

Positive results of a test for glucose are reported as trace and 1+ to 4+ when qualitative methods of testing are used, as is the case in routine analysis. Quantitative methods are used on 24-h

34   GUIDE TO DIAGNOSTIC PROCEDURES

samples and are reported as number of grams of glucose in the total 24-h urine output. Since the diabetic patient very often regulates the dosage of insulin in accordance with tests of his urine for glucose and since the nurse frequently performs the tests, it is important to know the methods used.

Two types of reactions are used in testing for glucose. One is reduction of a metallic ion (such as copper or bismuth) by glucose when heated, with a resulting precipitation and color change in the test material. The other is a color reaction, indicating the degree of positivity, based on the interaction of enzymes and glucose. In Benedict's test, Clinitest,[1] and Galatest,[2] the metallic ion is used. In Clinistix,[1], Urostix[1] and Testape,[3] the enzyme system is used.

The oldest method of testing for glucose in urine that is still used in some laboratories is Benedict's. Benedict's solution is an alkaline solution of copper sulfate (cupric ion), which, when heated in the presence of glucose, changes from blue to varying shades of orange to brick red, depending on the amount of cupric ion reduced to cuprous ion. As can be seen, this method is inconvenient for the patient or nurse testing the specimen, since heat is required to accomplish the reaction.

Clinitest tablets contain sodium hydroxide, which, when mixed with water, generates heat, thus providing the heat necessary for the reaction of glucose with the copper ion. With this method, the urine is added to a measured amount of water in a small test tube, and a tablet is dropped into the solution. The results are read as soon as the boiling has subsided.

With Clinistix, Urostix, or Testape, all that is necessary is to dip the test strip into the urine and read the color change according to the scale shown on the bottle or tape dispenser. The directions for performing this test must be followed meticulously because timing and care in handling the strips are critical to the accuracy of this method.

---

[1] Clinitest, Clinistix, and Urostix are products of the Ames Company, Elkhart, Ind.
[2] Galatest is the product of the Denver Chemical Manufacturing Co., New York.
[3] Testape is the product of E. R. Squibb & Sons, New York.

It is important that the choice of reagent used to detect the presence of glucose be known, since the sensitivity and specificity of the copper-reduction and enzyme methods are different (see Table 2-6). In choosing between the two methods, one must have in mind exactly the information being sought. Simply because the copper-reduction method is not specific for glucose does not rule out its being extremely useful, for there are occasions when detecting the presence of nonglucose reducing substances is of vital importance. A case in point would be the analysis of infant or child urines. Should the Clinitest be positive and the Clinistix negative, one must test further to identify the nonglucose reducing substance detected in the Clinitest. It may be galactose, in which case mental retardation could be a consequence of galactosemia that is not treated.

Since it is common practice to regulate insulin dosage on the basis of urine glucose levels, the choice of reagents becomes

TABLE 2-6   COMPARISON OF ENZYME AND COPPER-REDUCTION METHODS FOR DETECTION OF GLUCOSE

Reagent	Specificity	Sensitivity	False positives
Enzyme Clinistix Combistix Testape	Detects presence of glucose only	Reacts positively to as little as 0.1% glucose	Ascorbic acid; contamination with oxidizing agents
Copper ions Benedict's solution Clinitest tablets	Detects presence of glucose and other substances which reduce copper, e.g., galactose, lactose, fructose, maltose, salicylates, and certain drug metabolites	Reacts positively to 0.5% of the reducing substance	If test is for glucose only, any of the other compounds listed would give a false positive

important because of the differences in sensitivity. The enzyme method yields positive indications at lower levels of urinary glucose than those for the copper-reduction method.

Sources of error in the Clinistix method are primarily those of not following the directions meticulously and improper protection of the reagent strips from atmospheric and other contaminants. It is extremely important to keep the strips clean and dry. In using the Clinitest tablets, again one must follow the directions meticulously. Since the tablets are extremely hygroscopic, one must protect them from water from any source, including atmospheric air.

KETONE BODIES

Normal range: neg

In human physiology, the term *ketone bodies* refers to just three compounds: β-hydroxybutyric acid, acetoacetic (or diacetic) acid, and acetone, although there are many more ketone compounds known. These compounds are the products of fatty acid and fat metabolism. Ketones may be used by the body in lieu of the carbohydrates normally used for energy, and, in derangements of carbohydrate metabolism or intake, ketones are produced in considerable quantity. When this is excessive, ketosis develops, and ultimately acidosis, because of the exhaustion of the alkaline reserve of the body. Ketonuria is primarily associated with diabetic acidosis, although other conditions, such as starvation, ether anesthesia, and pernicious vomiting, can lead to this pathologic condition. In the laboratories, one of the most common methods of testing for acetone, the principal ketone and the one present in the greatest amount in most cases, is to mix a solution of sodium nitroprusside and urine and then overlay with ammonia, checking for a purple ring at the interface of the two liquids. However, powders have been perfected and put out commercially to test urine for acetone, and there is also a dip method, using a strip of paper impregnated with the reagent. In the latter two methods, a purple color indicates a positive test. The nurse may often be called upon to check the urine of the diabetic patient for acetone as well as for glucose.

BILIRUBIN, UROBILINOGEN, AND UROBILIN

Normal ranges
Bilirubin: none
Urobilinogen: 0.3–2.0 Ehrlich units/2 h or 1:8–1:16 titer
Urobilin: none

In older terminology, *bilirubin* is referred to as bile. However, with more complete understanding of the pathways of bilirubin metabolism and excretion, it is found that the pigment causing the characteristic color of urine in jaundice is bilirubin. Jaundice may be due to hapatocellular damage or obstruction, and differentiating between the two can be aided by tests for bilirubin and urobilinogen. Bilirubin is detected in the urine by qualitative methods. The simplest is inspection for the characteristic dark-amber color. When a urine specimen containing a considerable amount of bilirubin is shaken, foam produced has a yellow color. This is not true of amber colors due to other compounds in urine. Detection of small amounts of bilirubin in the urine preceding the manifestation of clinical jaundice is important is revealing latent and unsuspected liver disease. Free bilirubin (i.e., not conjugated with glucuronic acid or sulfates) is not water-soluble and therefore cannot be excreted in the urine.

Fouchet's test for bilirubin is dependent upon the production of a green color upon interaction of ferric chloride and bilirubin. A simple and sensitive test for bilirubin is done with Ictotest[1] tablets; the reaction is between bilazo compound and bilirubin and produces a purplish color, the degree of which corresponds to the amount of bilirubin. This test detects as little as 0.1 mg/dl urine, the lowest level at which bilirubin in the urine is abnormal.

Urobilinogen is produced in the intestinal tract by chemical reduction of the bilirubin excreted in the bile. This is accomplished by enteric bacteria normally present in the intestinal tract. Some of the urobilinogen is absorbed from the intestine and is carried back to the liver via the enterohepatic circulation to be excreted with bile. During this passage, small amounts of urobilinogen (1 percent of the total excreted) are excreted by the kidneys in the urine.

[1] Ictotest is the product of the Ames Company, Elkhart, Ind.

Two methods are used in testing the urine for urobilinogen: the Watson-Schwartz and Wallace-Diamond tests. In the former, the results are reported in Ehrlich units. One Ehrlich unit is equivalent to one milligram pure urobilinogen per one hundred milliliters solvent. The Wallace-Diamond method involves serial dilution of the urine prior to addition of the reagent, and results are reported as the titer, i.e., the highest dilution at which the reaction occurs.

Formerly, it was considered necessary to have a 24-h urine specimen for urobilinogen determinations, but this is being supplanted by a 2-h afternoon specimen. It has been found that maximal excretion of urobilinogen occurs from midafternoon to early evening. To carry out the 2-h test, the following procedure is used:

1. Have the patient empty his bladder at 2 P.M. and discard this sample. At 4 P.M., again have the patient empty his bladder completely. Save the entire specimen and send it to the laboratory without delay.
2. If the patient voids before 4 P.M., save the specimen, label it with the time collected, and send it to the laboratory without delay. In this case, the 4 P.M. collection is not necessary.

The nurse's responsibility in this test is to be sure to note the total time during which collection was made and to make sure that the entire specimen is sent to the laboratory, since the volume of specimen is critical in determining the results. For the 24-h specimen, it is necessary to collect all the urine voided in a 24-h period. This is done according to the following procedure:

1. Have the patient void at 8 A.M., discard this sample, and then save all urine voided within the next 24 h, completing the period by having him void for the last time at 8 A.M. the day following the start of collection.
2. Caution the patient to save his urine before defecating. Collect the specimen in a large brown bottle, and add ½ teaspoon crystals of sodium carbonate and a few milliliters of petroleum ether as preservative.

TABLE 2-7   BILIRUBIN: PATHWAYS AND MECHANISMS
OF METABOLISM

Event	Site	Product	Color
RBC destruction	Reticuloendothelial system	Free hemo-globin	Red
Hemoglobin breakdown	Reticuloendothelial system	Bilirubin	Reddish-orange
Bilirubin conjugation	Liver	Bilirubin glucuride or sulfate	No change
Bilirubin glucuronide reduction by bacteria	Intestine	Urobilinogen	Colorless
Urobilinogen absorption	Enterohepatic circulation	No change	No change
Urobilinogen oxidation by bacteria	Intestine	Urobilin	Dark brown

Urobilin is the product of bacterial oxidation of urobilinogen during its passage through the intestinal tract. Urobilin is dark brown, accounting for much of the normal color of feces. Since the formation of urobilin is dependent upon bacterial action, none is present in the urine when freshly voided. Only upon bacterial contamination of urine having elevated levels of urobilinogen is urobilin formed. This is the rationale behind insistence on freshly voided specimens for urobilinogen determinations. No tests for urobilin are done.

PORPHYRINS

Normal range: trace (17–99 µg/24 h)

Coproporphyrinuria may be present in liver disease, but the principal diseases producing porphyrinuria are both congenital and are probably due to an inherent error of metabolism. *Congenital porphyria* may be detected in the early years. It is manifested by a pinkish-brown staining of the teeth and bones. The urine of patients with this disease is usually pinkish-yellow to reddish-black, and it becomes darker as it stands in sunlight. An outstanding clinical feature is development of severe skin lesions in those parts of the body which are exposed to sunlight. *Acute porphyria* (Hoffman prefers the designation *acute intermittent porphyria)* is seen in adults. Although the patient may consistently excrete porphyrins in excess of the normal level, it is not usually noted until there is an acute attack, at which time the urine becomes deep red. The acute phase is marked by severe abdominal pain, neuropathy (frequently with paralysis), and mental disturbances. The abdominal pain is severe enough to simulate conditions requiring surgical treatment. Like the other form of porphyria, acute porphyria is a congenital disease. A single fresh urine specimen is usually called for in a test for porphyrins, although a 24-h specimen may be indicated.

OCCULT BLOOD

The term "occult" refers to that which is hidden. Ordinarily, one might suppose that red blood cells would easily be detected by microscopic examination. However, the sensitivity of the microscopic examination is less than that of chemical detection.

Microscopic Examination of the Urine

GENERAL CONSIDERATIONS

Other than percutaneous renal biopsy, there can be no more valuable examination than microscopic evaluation of the urinary sediment. It mirrors characteristic elements found in infection, collagen and allied diseases causing glomerulitis, nephrotic syndrome, acute tubular necrosis, and advanced chronic renal disease. To obtain the urine sediment for study, the specimen is centrifuged, the supernatant fluid poured off, and sediment then resuspended in the remaining liquid. A drop of this material is then examined, unstained and, when indicated, with Sternheimer-Malbin stain.

CELLULAR ELEMENTS

Epithelial Cells

Renal cells are small, round, polyhedral cells with a single, relatively large nucleus. In hemochromatosis, renal infarction, or chronic passive congestion, they may contain hemosiderin. Their presence in the sediment is an index of renal damage.

Transitional cells are two to three times the size of renal cells, and their forms may be pear, spindle, or round with tail-like processes (caudate) in shape. They originate from the lining of the pelvises, ureters, and bladder. They are present when pathologic conditions exist in these areas.

Squamous cells originate from the superficial layers of the urethra and vagina. They are large, flat, thin, and have a single small nucleus. Their presence in the urine is not indicative of a pathologic condition, since they are normally sloughed from time to time.

Epithelial cells are reported as number per low-power field or, when too numerous to count, from 1+ to 4+.

White Blood Cells

These may be reported as *"WBC"* or *"pus cells."* Normally, not more than four cells per high-power field are seen. An excess of this number is considered indicative of an inflammatory process somewhere in the urinary tract. In any question of pyuria in women, a "clean-catch" specimen is necessary to rule out vaginal contamination of the specimen (see page 21 for collection of a clean-voided specimen). When the Sternheimer-Malbin stain is used in the microscopic preparation, two types of white blood cells may be seen. In one, the nucleus and cytoplasm are contracted, and the nucleus heavily stained. Larger cells, with very pale-staining nuclei and notable Brownian movement of cytoplasmic inclusions, are known as "glitter cells." There are many such cells present in pyelonephritis.

Red Blood Cells

These are reported as *RBC*. Normally, no more than an occasional red blood cell per high-power field is seen. When red blood cells have lost their hemoglobin content but remain intact, they may be referred to as "ghost cells" and reported as such. Again, in women, it is necessary to rule out vaginal contamination as a source of red blood cells in the urine.

Red blood cells can be found in almost any disease of the kidney or urinary tract. It is obviously important to determine the source of hemorrhage and to determine whether it is acute or chronic, gross or microscopic. This is aided by clinical findings and by accompanying structures, such as casts or epithelial cells, in the urine sediment. As was noted in the discussion of pH and specific gravity, it is important to recognize the fact that red blood cells may be hemolyzed. It is in such cases that tests for occult blood are especially valuable.

CASTS

Casts are molds of the tubules within which they form, and are made up of plasma-protein gel and/or cells. In order for the casts of form, there must be a pH of 6.0 or less and a high salt concentration in the glomerular filtrate. Normally, no casts are seen in the urine. When they do appear, they are reported as the number seen per low-power field. There are three types of casts: hyaline, epithelial, and blood. Each is named for the predominant element contained in it. As epithelial casts age within the tubules, they become *granular* owing to degeneration of the cells which make up the cast. These are referred to as granular casts and are further described as finely or coarsely granular.

The importance of recognizing types of casts cannot be overemphasized, since they are extremely important in diagnosing the location of hemorrhagic or inflammatory sites. Obviously, the presence of blood casts indicates that the site of hemorrhage is within the renal system itself rather than in the lower urinary tract. The same may be said of the location of inflammatory disease through the recognition of white blood cell casts.

Significance

Hyaline casts are seen in intrinsic renal disease, heart failure, shock, fever, and excessive exercise. When red blood cells are noted within them, bleeding through damaged glomerular capillaries or ruptured tubular walls may be suspected. When white blood cells are noted in the casts, infection within the kidney is indicated, and these are associated with pyelonephritis. Distinction of cellular content of casts is important in the differential diagnosis of renal or lower-urinary-tract disease.

Red blood cell casts are the product of glomerular-capillary changes in glomerulitis which permit the escape of cells and fibrinogen into Bowman's capsular space. In the upper part of the tubule, the cells become tightly packed in a fibrin clot. When the casts are fresh, outlines of the cells are readily seen; then cells disintegrate, and the cast has a homogeneous red-orange appearance. This is a true blood cast. These casts are seen, for example, in glomerulonephritis and lupus nephritis.

White blood cell casts are formed of cells and fibrin in a high concentration of tubular contents. When these casts are fresh, clumps of cells are seen in the fibrin mesh; then, as the cast ages, outlines are lost, and finely granular morphology is assumed. These casts are seen in acute exacerbations of pyelonephritis.

Tubular-cell casts are aggregates of sloughed epithelial cells. As noted above, they may degenerate to *coarsely granular, finely granular*, and, finally, *waxy* morphology. These casts, in acute tubular necrosis, contain free hemoglobin, which gives them a reddish tinge. Acute tubular damage, such as in heavy-metal poisoning, advanced glomerulonephritis, pyelonephritis, and malignant nephrosclerosis, may be characterized by this type of cast. *Broad granular* casts, also called renal-failure casts, are formed in the dilated tubules of advanced renal insufficiency. Their presence indicates a grave prognosis.

FAT BODIES

In nephrotic syndromes, tubule cells are characteristically engorged with fat; when they slough off singly into the lumen of the tubule, they are oval *fat bodies.* They measure 20 to 50 μm and have varying sizes of fat droplets in large amounts. When they coalesce, *fatty casts* are formed. "Lipiduria" refers to the presence of any of these fatty elements in the urine.

TELESCOPED SEDIMENT

When urinary sediment contains all varieties of casts and cells, it is known as *telescoped sediment,* since it combines all the ages of these elements. This type of sediment is seen particularly in lupus nephritis and periateritis.

CRYSTALS

Only crystals of administered drugs, such as sulfonamides, or those of protein breakdown, such as leucine or tyrosine, are significant per se. Where there is a tendency to form renal calculi, the predominant type of crystals present should be noted.

Crystals commonly seen in acid urine are amorphous urates, uric acid, and calcium oxalate crystals. Those commonly seen in alkaline urine are amorphous phosphates, triple phosphate, calcium diphosphate, and ammonium biurate crystals.

MISCELLANEOUS FORMED ELEMENTS

Cotton fibers, wood fibers, etc., may be seen in the urine sediment and are of no significance.

Normally there are no bacteria in urine, but after it passes through the urethra and is contaminated by the secretions of accessory structures, bacteria may be present. In urinary-tract infections, the presence of bacteria is, of course, significant and should be noted.

Occasionally, spermatozoa may be seen in the urine. This is not significant in itself, but it should be reported in order to account for any positive test for protein that might have resulted.

In trichomoniasis, the parasite (*Trichomonas vaginalis*) may be present in the urine. This is due to contamination from vaginal secretions, but it should be reported, since it may be the first indication that the disease is present. Although it is thought that there are few, if any, cases of trichomoniasis in men, it is not out of the realm of possibility that trichomonads might be reported seen in a urine specimen from a man.

ADDIS COUNT

Thomas Addis devised a method of studying a 12- (or 24-) h urinary output as a diagnostic and prognostic aid in treatment of renal disease. Table 2-8 indicates the Addis interpretations of white and red blood cell and cast counts.

Procedures

For this test, the patient is allowed no fluids during the test period, and he collects all the urine excreted during the prescribed period. The volume of the output is measured, and a quantitative determination of protein is done. The sediment from a measured amount is examined, and accurate counts of the number of each of the cellular elements are made. If the recommended 12-h collection is not possible, approximation of the Addis count can be made with

TABLE 2-8   NORMAL AND PATHOLOGIC FINDINGS IN ADDIS
SEDIMENT COUNTS

Condition	RBC/mm^3	WBC/mm^3	$Casts/mm^3$
Normal	0–5,000	0–500,000	1,000,000
Acute nephritis	690,000	405,000,000	48,000,000
Chronic nephritis			
Active	1,850,000	34,000,000	14,000,000
Latent	48,000	16,000,000	2,000,000
Terminal nephritis	348,000	26,400,000	10,000,000

SOURCE: From Opal Helper, "Manual of Clinical Laboratory Methods," 4th ed., 1954. Used with permission of Charles C Thomas, Publisher, Springfield, Ill.

the first morning urine passed (if the patient has not taken fluids for 16 h prior to voiding the morning sample). The normal output in total volume during the Addis count test period is 8 to 16 dl. The diurnal output is three to four times the volume of the nocturnal output.

Collection of Specimens

Aside from the restriction on fluids, no changes are made in the patient's routine when the collection is being made for the Addis count. The nurse may instruct the patient about collection of the specimen as follows:

1. Have the patient collect the specimen in two bottles, each of which has been rinsed with a little Formalin solution in order to preserve the cellular elements. One bottle is used for the daytime 12-h period and the other for the night period.
2. Have the patient void at 8 A.M., discard this sample, and save all urine voided within the next 12-h period for the diurnal specimen. At 8 P.M., he uses the second bottle to collect all urine voided from that time until 8 A.M. the following morning.
3. Keep the bottles of specimen cold in order to prevent bacterial growth.
4. Instruct the patient to save urine before defecating.

AMINOACIDURIAS

The disorders characterized by the presence of increased amounts of amino acids in the blood and urine may be due to an inborn error of metabolism,[1] severe liver disease, or the results of a disorder of tubular transport mechanisms. The metabolic-error type is also termed "overflow aminoaciduria." The association of mental retardation as an effect of the accumulation of excessive amounts of amino acids has focused attention of early diagnosis and intervention to lessen or prevent damage. Identification of the amino acids requires analysis by chromatography. The ferric chloride

[1] First described by Archibald Garrod in his early studies of genetics.

screening test may be used in some instances as a general indication of aminoaciduria.

Of all the kinds of aminoacidurias, phenylketonuria has received the most attention, leading to the mandatory requirement, in some states, for screening newborns. Two methods are available for screening urine specimens for *phenylalanine:* ferric chloride and Phenistix.[1] In the ferric chloride test, 5 ml of urine is required, and there are a number of substances which may give false positives. The Phenistix method uses a different reagent source of ferric ions, requires nothing more than a urine-wet diaper for test material, and is not subject to the many interfering substances producing false positives. Careful attention to the procedure using Phenistix is essential, but it is a simple procedure. The stick is moistened by being dipped into a specimen or pressed against a wet diaper. A positive screening test must be followed up by definitive tests before the diagnosis of phenylketonuria may be made. Three important criteria must be met in making this diagnosis. There must be serum phenylalanine levels at or above 20 mg/dl on at least two occasions; serum tyrosine levels must be no higher than 5 mg/dl in the same serum samples; and high concentrations of phenylalanine metabolites such as o-hydroxyphenylacetic acid must be present in the urine.

CATECHOLAMINES

Epinephrine (adrenaline) and norepinephrine (noradrenaline), classified as catecholamines, are secreted by the adrenal medulla and by some rare tumors. As will be readily recognized, these compounds have a marked effect on the blood pressure through the effect of norepinephrine on the peripheral arteries and that of epinephrine on the cardiac output, both resulting in increased blood pressure. In patients having otherwise unexplained hypertension, tests for catecholamines (or their metabolites) are used to diagnose presence of tumors which secrete these compounds. Tumors associated with elevated levels of catecholamines and their metabolites [primarily homovanillic acid (4-hydroxy-3-methoxy-

<hr>

[1] Product of Ames Company, Elkhart, Ind.

TABLE 2-9 AMINOACIDURIAS

Disease	Elevated amino acids (serum)	Abnormal enzymes	Screening-test reaction	Clinical features
Overflow				
Phenylketonuria	Phenylalanine	Phenylalanine hydroxylase	Green	Mental retardation, fits, eczema, fair hair
Tyrosinosis	Tyrosine	p-Hydroxyphenyl-pyruvic acid	Quick-fading green	Hepatic cirrhosis, Fanconi syndrome, renal glycosuria, renal rickets
Histidemia	Histidine	Histidase	Olive	Mild or severe mental retardation
Maple syrup urine disease	Leucine, valine, isoleucine, alloisoleucine	Branched-chain keto acid decarboxylase	Blue	Vomiting, hypertonicity, severe mental retardation, early death
Hypervalinemia	Valine	Valine alpha-keto isovaleric acid transaminase		Mental retardation
Hyperglycinemia	Glycine	Not known		Periodic vomiting, lethargy, ketosis, osteoporosis, mental retardation
Citrullinemia	Citrulline	Argininosuccinic acid synthesase		Mental retardation, liver disease
Hyperlysinemia	Lysine	Not known		Mental retardation, fits

Hyperprolinemia			
Type I	Proline	Proline oxidase	Mental retardation, fits
Type II	Proline	Δ'-pyrroline-5-carboxlylate dehydrogenase	Mental retardation, fits
Homocystinuria	Methionine, homocystine	Cystathionine synthetase	Mental retardation, dislocated lenses, vascular accidents, Marfanlike syndrome, osteoporosis
Alkaptonuria	Homogentisic acid (no abnormal amino acid)	Homogentisic acid oxidase	Usually asymptomatic until middle life; ochronosis; urine becomes pink, then black on standing
Argininosuccinic aciduria	Argininosuccinic acid	Argininosuccinase	Mental retardation, ataxia, ammonia intoxication
Cystathioninuria	Cystathionine	Cystathioninase	Mental retardation, congenital acidosis, thrombocytopenia, pituitary gland abnormalities
Homocystinuria	Homocystine	Cystathionine synthetase	See above
Renal-transport disorder			
Cystinuria	Cystine, lysine arginine, ornithine		Hypophosphatemic rickets, glycosuria, deposition of cystine crystals

SOURCE: Adapted from Kodak CHROMATO/O/SCREEN Analysis Kit for Amino Acids, publication J J-172, Eastman Kodak Company, Rochester, N. Y. 1971.

phenylacetic acid) and vanilmandelic acid (4-hydroxy-3-methoxy-mandelic acid)] include pheochromocytoma, ganglioneuroma, neuroblastoma, and ganglioneuroblastoma. In carcinoid syndrome, 5-hydroxyindoleacetic acid (5-HIAA) is increased. Normal values for these compounds are as follows:

Catecholamines	Less than 14 μg/dl
Homovanillic acid (HVA)	Less than 15 mg/24 h
Vanilmandelic acid (VMA)	0.5–7.0 mg/24 h
5-Hydroxyindoleacetic acid (5-HIAA)	Less than 15 mg/24 h

If the patient is not consistently hypertensive, urine should be obtained during a period of stress or hypertension for catecholamine determinations. If there is persistent hypertension, however, a single voiding of a random sample may be used. Catecholamines are unstable, and the test should be done as soon after the collection as possible. The specimen may be preserved in a special preservative if delay is unavoidable.

VMA is excreted in larger amounts than catecholamines are, making it possible to achieve greater accuracy in the determination. It is a more stable compound, and fewer technical problems are involved in the procedure. A 24-h specimen is required, using hydrochloric acid as preservative (to maintain a pH of 3.0), and collected in a brown bottle. Prior to collection, the patient's diet is restricted by elimination of coffee, tea, chocolate, and bananas for 2 days. Since drugs may also interfere with the test, medications are also discontinued for 2 days prior to beginning, and during, the collection period. Similar precautions are required for HVA determinations. A random sample is satisfactory for 5-HIAA analysis.

CHORIONIC GONADOTROPIC HORMONE

The usual test for human chorionic gonadotropic hormone (HCG), the compound present in pregnancy and certain tumors, is qualitative, determining only the presence or absence of the hormone. However, with the development of tests based on principles of immunologic reactions, quantitative results, reported as titers, can

be obtained. The tumors which produce HCG include hydatidiform mole, choriocarcinoma, and testicular teratoma. In pregnancy,
the tests are usually positive by the tenth to fourteenth day after
the first missed menstrual period. Peak levels of the HCG are
present in the first trimester of pregnancy, declining perceptibly
after the fourteenth week of gestation.

HCG is a glycoprotein, and this makes it possible to use principles of immunology for testing for its presence. The reagents required are anti-HCG serum (prepared commercially) and sensitized
sheep red blood cells or latex particles. The red blood cells or
latex particles provide the indicator to determine whether there
has been an antigen-antibody reaction between the HCG present in
(or absent from) the urine or blood serum of the patient and the
anti-HCG reagent. The following chart shows the possible reactions
and the corresponding results:

	STEP I	STEP II		
Antibody	Unknown sample containing	Antigen indicator	Reaction	Result
Anti-HCG serum	HCG	Sensitized RBC or HCG-coated latex	Neutralization of antiserum; no agglutination	Pos
Anti-HCG serum	No HCG	As above	No neutraliza-tion; aggluti-nation present	Neg

Significance

Tests for HCG are important for a number of conditions.
Combining the physician's knowledge of clinical findings and the
test results, it is possible to make differential diagnoses as follows:

1. Evaluation of amenorrhea or hemorrhage during the meno-
   pausal period; diagnosis of uterine tumors, such as myofibromas,
   and malignancies that cause uterine enlargement simulating
   that of pregnancy.
2. Evaluation of the viability of possible or known pregnancy in

which there is vaginal bleeding. In known pregnancy, the test aids in determining partial or missed abortion, since death of the fetus and placenta precludes presence of HCG. The test is frequently used to aid decisions involving possible surgical intervention.
3. Diagnosis of rare malignancies that secrete HCG: hydatidiform mole, choriocarcinoma, and testicular teratoma.

Collection of Specimens for HCG Tests

Blood serum may be used for the test, and the blood for this purpose may be drawn at any time during the day. Sufficient blood should be obtained to yield at least 1.5 ml serum. When urine is used as test material, the patient is instructed to avoid all fluid intake after the evening meal, in order that the first urine voided the following morning will be well concentrated. At least 2 oz urine are required for the test. The specimen should be delivered to the laboratory as soon as possible after collection.

RENAL CALCULI

The incidence of renal calculi has been estimated at about 10 cases per 10,000 population per year, based on hospital admissions with this diagnosis. Stone analysis to determine the components can be useful in directing diagnosis of predisposing diseases or conditions and in providing prevention of recurrence by appropriate regimens. The conditions leading to stone formation are varied, and probably not all have been identified. Precipitation or con-glomeration of mucopolysaccharides and mucoproteins to form a nidus or matrix upon which crystal-forming components of the urine may build up is a precondition to stone formation. Foreign bodies, urine stasis, as well as infection, also have been implicated. Table 2-10 shows the conditions associated with various types of renal calculi, and Table 2-11 relates gross appearance of calculi to their composition. Composition of stones is determined by chemical analysis, microscopy with polarized light, x-ray diffraction, and infrared spectroscopy.

TABLE 2-10
CONDITIONS ASSOCIATED WITH RENAL-CALCULI FORMATION

Type of calculus	Associated condition
Calcium	Idiopathic hypercalcemia Primary hyperparathyroidism Bone disease (e.g., osteoporosis) Excessive milk, alkali, or vitamin D intake Renal-tubular-acidosis syndrome Sarcoidosis Berylliosis
Calcium oxaluria	Oxaluria Incomplete catabolism of carbohydrates Isohydria at pH 5.5 to 6.0
Calcium phosphate	Isohydria at pH 7.0 or higher Infection with urea-splitting bacteria
Uric acid/urates	Gout Polycythemia Leukemia Lymphoma Liver disease Isohydria at pH 5.0 or lower
Cystine	Transient acute phases of chronic renal diseases such as pyelonephritis Heavy metal toxicity Aminoaciduria Renal-tubular-acidosis syndrome

SOURCE: Adapted from J. A. Freeman and M. F. Beeler, "Laboratory Medicine—Clinical Microscopy," pp. 126–131, Lea & Febiger, Philadelphia, 1974.

TABLE 2-11   CORRELATION OF GROSS APPEARANCE
OF RENAL CALCULI WITH CHEMICAL COMPOSITION

Gross appearance	Probable component(s)
Staghorn	Magnesium ammonium phosphate, cystine
Mulberry or jackstone (often very hard, with sharp edges, black surface)	Oxalate
White, or light colored; friable; concentric-ring formation on cut surface	Calcium phosphate complexes (hydroxyl or carbonate apatites)
Smooth, waxy	Cystine
Yellow, ochre	Uric acid

NOTE: Various combinations of constituent compounds may be found on analysis.
SOURCE: Adapted from J. A. Freeman and M. F. Beeler, "Laboratory Medicine—Clinical Microscopy," p. 98, Lea & Febiger, Philadelphia, 1974.

TABLE 2-12   SUMMARY OF COMMON URINALYSIS FINDINGS

Test	Condition	Test results	Required specimen
Specific gravity	1. Diabetes mellitus	1. Greater than 1.030 when glucose is present in high concentration	1. Random
	2. Diabetes insipidus	2. Less than 1.010	2. Random

	3. Kidney damage
	   a. Renal shutdown
	   b. Nephrosis
		3. Less than 1.010	3. Random or indicated for concentration-dilution test

Protein	1. Nephritis 2. Nephrosis 3. Renal calculi 4. Toxemia of pregnancy	1–5. All positive in varying degrees, depending on the extent of damage	1–5. Random on 24-h specimen, as directed

TABLE 2-12   (continued)

Test	Condition	Test results	Required specimen
	5. Inflammatory disease of some portion of the genitourinary system		
	6. Multiple myeloma	6. Bence Jones positive	6. Random
	7. Orthostatic proteinuria	7. Positive after exercise	7. As directed by the laboratory
Glucose	1. Diabetes mellitus	1. Positive when blood glucose level is elevated	1. Random or as directed in relation to meals
	2. Low renal threshold	2. Positive despite normal blood glucose levels	2. Random
	3. Head injury	3. May be positive despite normal blood glucose level	3. Random
	4. Adrenocorticotropic hormone (ACTH) therapy	4. May be positive and is transitory	4. Random
Ketone bodies (acetone and diacetic acid)	1. Diabetic acidosis	1. Positive	All random
	2. Ether anesthesia	2. Positive (transitory)	
	3. Starvation	3. Positive	
	4. Pernicious vomiting	4. Positive	
Bilirubin, urobilinogen, urobilin	1. Hepatic disease	1. Positive	All random or as directed for special periods
	2. Hemolytic disease a. Congenital b. Acquired c. Posthemolytic transfusion reaction	2. Positive	

TABLE 2-12   (continued)

Test	Condition	Test results	Required specimen
Porphyrins	1. Congenital porphyria	1. Positive	All random
	2. Acute porphyria	2. Positive	
Microscopic	1. Inflammatory processes	1. WBC numerous; RBC may be present; bacteria may be present	All specimens in this group may be collected at random
	2. Nephritis	2. RBC numerous; casts numerous	
	3. Nephrosis	3. RBC may be numerous; casts may be present	
	4. Insufficient hydration during sulfonamide therapy	4. Characteristic sulfonamide crystals	
	5. Trichomoniasis	5. *Trichomonas* present (in women, *T. vaginalis* may be present in the urine incidental to vaginal contamination)	
	6. Schistosomiasis	6. RBC numerous; ova of *Schistosoma haematobium* may be found	
	7. Renal calculi	7. RBC present in varying numbers	
	8. Malignant conditions	8. RBC in varying numbers	
	9. Tuberculosis of urinary system	9. RBC in varying numbers, WBC in varying numbers	

REFERENCES

Davidsohn, Israel, and John B. Henry (eds.): "Todd-Sanford Clinical Diagnosis by Laboratory Methods," 15th ed., Saunders, Philadelphia, 1974.

Freeman, J. A., and M. F. Beeler: "Laboratory Medicine—Clinical Microscopy," Lea & Febiger, Philadelphia, 1974.

Lippman, R. W.: "Urine and Urinary Sediment. A Practical Manual and Atlas," Charles C Thomas, Springfield, Ill., 1951.

Mainwaring, Catherine: Clean Voided Specimens for Mass Screening, *Amer. J. Nurs.,* **61**(11):67 1961.

"Modern Urinalysis. A Guide to the Diagnosis of Urinary Tract Diseases and Metabolic Disorders," Ames Company, Division of Miles Laboratories, Inc., Elkhart, Ind., 1973.

Nora, James J., and F. Clarke Fraser: "Medical Genetics: Principles and Practice," Lea & Febiger, Philadelphia, 1974.

Oser, B. L. (ed.): "Hawk's Practical Physiological Chemistry," 14th ed., McGraw-Hill, New York, 1965.

Rubini, M. E., and A. V. Wolf: Refractometric Determination of Total Solids and Water of Serum and Urine, *J. Biol. Chem.* **225**: 869, 1957.

Searcy, Ronald L.: "Diagnostic Biochemistry," McGraw-Hill, New York, 1969.

Sullivan, Lawrence P.: "Physiology of the Kidney," Lea & Febiger, Philadelphia, 1974.

Tietz, N. W., (ed.): "Fundamentals of Clinical Chemistry," Saunders, Philadelphia, 1970.

"Urodynamics. Concepts Relating to Urinalysis," Ames Company, Division of Miles Laboratories, Elkhart, Inc., 1974.

THREE

HEMATOLOGIC EXAMINATIONS

Nearly all hematologic examinations may be done on capillary blood, i.e., blood taken from a finger prick, but many times, when performed in conjunction with other tests requiring more blood, venous blood is used. Nurses and technologists must keep in mind the fact that the patient may be undergoing venipuncture for the first time and may be quite apprehensive about it. It is easy for nurses and technologists to forget (or ignore) this fact, and the patient may sense the apparent heartlessness, which increases his apprehension. We know that the procedure is simple and need not be painful if done correctly, with the patient's cooperation. Consequently, a calm and sympathetic explanation of the procedure can help the patient overcome his apprehension and give him confidence in the person performing the venipuncture. Aside from the actual physical discomfort of a venipuncture, the patient may well have questions concerning the implications of the tests to be done. The patient may be informed that many different tests may be performed on blood drawn from the vein. It may be well to explain to the patient which tests are being done for him, although whether he should be told will depend on the individual case and the doctor in charge.

Another common fear of patients when blood is drawn from the vein is that a great amount of blood is being taken. For the usual tests, not more than 10 ml are ordinarily required. This should be translated into terms understood by the patient, since he can probably comprehend amounts better in terms of tablespoons rather than milliliters. He should be assured that this is not an excessive amount of blood to lose. Another way to assure the patient that he is not losing too much blood is to inform him of the total amount of blood the average person has circulating in his body: between 5 and 6 qt. Also reassuring is the fact that 50 ml of blood is manufactured every day in the normal person as part of the normal course of physiology of blood replacement, whether he loses any blood or not.

It seems a common thing for the patient to be horrified at the sight of someone deliberately taking "so much blood." When it is his own life's fluid, every little drop is extremely precious; hence it is necessary to assure him that he can bear the loss. There may be times, of course, when more than 10 ml of blood may be needed for multiple tests. In this case, it is even more important that the patient be assured that the amount of blood taken will not harm him.

PROCEDURE FOR VENIPUNCTURE

1. Equipment
   a. Tourniquet
   b. Sharp hypodermic needle (gauge 20 to 23, choice depending on the amount of blood needed or the infusion to be given and the size of the patient's vein)
   c. Alcohol sponge

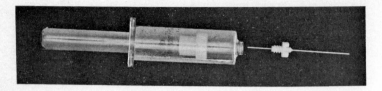

FIG. 3-1 The Vacutainer system.

    d. Dry cotton ball

    e. Clean, dry syringe or Vacutainer[1] adapter and tube (see Fig. 3-1)

2. Method

    a. The usual veins of choice for venipuncture are those in the antecubital area, the median basilic being the best. Those at the sides of the arm tend to roll away from the needle point.

    b. Instruct the patient to hold his arm straight and stiff.

    c. Apply the tourniquet just above the elbow.

    d. Instruct the patient to close his hand in a tight fist. If the veins do not distend rather quickly, it is helpful to have the patient open and close his hand several times.

    e. If the vein is not obvious, palpate the area for the vein, since it may be felt even though it is not seen. There is a firmness but resilience in the distended vein.

    f. Swab the area of the puncture with the alcohol sponge.

    g. Hold the skin below the site of puncture taut by pulling the skin down with the thumb of the free hand.

    h. Syringe procedure: Insert the needle, bevel up, with a quick one-two motion so that it enters the skin and then the vein. When the needle point enters the lumen of the vein, blood comes into the tip of the syringe. Draw the sample by gently pulling back on the plunger. Release the tourniquet and withdraw the needle. Place a dry piece of cotton over the puncture site and hold firmly for a few minutes in order to prevent leakage of blood into the cutaneous tissue surrounding the puncture site. Vacutainer procedure: Select the appropriate

[1] Vacutainer is a product of Beckton-Dickson Co., Rutherford, N.J.

tube[1] for specimen desired and insert into adapter so that the stopper rests on the point of the internal needle. Insert the external needle, bevel up, with a quick one-two motion so that it enters the skin and then the vein. Push on the bottom of the tube so that the internal needle pierces the diaphragm of the stopper and enters the tube. The tube will fill to the maximum allowed by the vacuum present. Multiple tubes of blood may be obtained by disengaging the filled tube and replacing it with another, while keeping the needle in the vein. To minimize leakage of blood into the adapter, the needle may be gently held up against the wall of the vein to occlude the bevel while the transfer is accomplished. When appropriate amounts of blood have been obtained, release the tourniquet and withdraw the needle. Place a dry piece of cotton over the puncture site and hold firmly for a few minutes to prevent leakage of blood into the cutaneous tissue surrounding the puncture site.

EXAMINATION OF THE BONE MARROW

General Considerations

The most valuable source of information for diagnosis and prognosis of the blood dyscrasias is the bone marrow, since it is in the red bone marrow that blood cells are formed. In total volume, the bone marrow constitutes the most extensive tissue in the body. In adults, the most easily available supplies of bone marrow for study are the sternum and the iliac crest. Since it is a surgical procedure and requires delicate skill, the puncture must be performed by a doctor, usually the pathologist.

The patient may well be upset at the prospect of a marrow puncture, both because of what may be revealed by the studies and because of the discomfort of the procedure itself. The pain involved in obtaining bone marrow is ordinarily not too great, since the skin

---

[1] Specimen tubes from which air has been evacuated, creating a vacuum, are available with color-coded stoppers. The color of the stopper indicates the type of anticoagulant, if any, present.

and periosteum are anesthetized before the needle for aspiration is introduced. The most marked discomfort occurs when the aspiration itself is done. Almost invariably, the patient gasps a little with pain, which is caused by the negative pressure produced when the plunger of the syringe is pulled back.

It may be disconcerting to the patient to have a number of persons accompany the doctor who is to perform the aspiration. Ordinarily the pathologist will have a technologist to take care of the material obtained and sometimes a nurse, who assists him with the surgical procedure. Often, however, there may be student observers learning about the procedure. The patient may need assurance that the procedure is a simple one, which should not upset him unduly.

Procedure for Marrow Puncture and Aspiration

1. Materials
    a. Sterile tray with
        (1) Drape towels
        (2) 2- and 10-ml syringes
        (3) 25-gauge needle
        (4) Sternal needle
        (5) Tincture of Merthiolate
        (6) 1% Novocain
        (7) Small bandage
        (8) Collodion
    b. Laboratory supplies
        (1) Glass slides and cover slips
        (2) Test tubes, plain and heparinized
2. Method
    a. If the patient is apprehensive, a sedative may be given ½ h before the procedure is scheduled to be done.
    b. Prepare the skin over the puncture site by shaving (if necessary) and cleaning with Merthiolate. Drape sterile towels around the selected site. Infiltrate the skin with the anesthetic, and then insert the needle deeper in order to anesthetize the periosteum.

c. Introduce the sternal needle. As the cortex is reached, it is necessary to push the needle with a boring motion to penetrate into the marrow space. There is obvious lack of resistance to the needle when this space is reached. The marrow cavity is usually 5 to 15 mm in depth. The sternal needle is equipped with a guard to prevent penetration to any dangerous depth.

d. When the marrow cavity is reached, remove the stylet from the needle and attach a sterile 10-ml syringe. Aspirate about 1 to 2 ml material and hand it to the technologist, who makes the smears, etc.

e. Replace the stylet in the needle and withdraw the needle. Close the puncture site with collodion and apply a small dressing.

Interpretation of Cells Present in Bone Marrow

Direct smears of the marrow are made immediately. Some of the material maybe placed in a tube containing heparin to prevent clotting, and the remainder is allowed to clot. In studying the bone-marrow preparations, the hematologist inspects the smears for the presence of abnormal cells, the proportion of cells of both the erythroid and the myeloid series, and the characteristics of the predominant type of cell. A count is made of the nucleated cells in order to obtain a definite idea of the percentage of each type of cell present. Depending upon the disease suspected, a statement is then made as to the presence or absence of the cells that are characteristic of the type of disease suspected. Bone-marrow studies are not considered diagnostic in themselves, but when they are part of the clinician's overall evaluation, they are a most valuable aid. The blood cells are seen in all stages of development, from the most immature to those ready for release into the peripheral circulation. When the marrow is hyperplastic, with a predominance of a particular cell in a series, such as myelocyte, myelocytic leukemia may be diagnosed. On the other hand, when the marrow is hypoplastic, there is a lack of cell production and a disease such as aplastic anemia may be diagnosed. When the cell development is arrested at a given level of maturation, as seen in pernicious anemia, the diagnosis is made from this finding in conjunction with the clinical findings.

BLOOD VOLUME

In order to determine the proportion of blood to total body weight, a blood-volume study may be done. This is accomplished by determining the red blood cell or plasma volume and then calculating the total blood volume. Plasma volume may be measured by injecting a dye (Evans blue) into the blood stream and, after allowing sufficient time for complete dilution of the dye in the blood, determining the precise degree of dilution, thus obtaining information from which to calculate total volume. With the development of the use of radionuclides, radioactive chromium is now also used to determine red blood cell volume (see Chap. 12).

Procedure

A blood sample is drawn from the patient, with strict sterile conditions maintained, and the red cells of the sample are treated, i.e., tagged with radioactive sodium chromate, and reintroduced into the patient's bloodstream. At given intervals, samples are obtained and hematocrit and radioactivity counts made to determine the dilution of the radioactive blood cells. The principle of these tests is that total volume may be determined by finding the degree of dilution of a solution or, in the case of ^{51}Cr, of radioactivity when the solution or radioactive material is mixed with an unknown volume of another solution.

Preparation of the Patient

This procedure requires at least two venipunctures for the dye test. The process requires about 1½ h to complete.

1. The patient must be completely at rest. The test is best done before the morning meal.

TABLE 3-1   NORMAL PLASMA, ERYTHROCYTE,
AND TOTAL BLOOD VOLUMES

(ml/kg body weight)

Sex	Plasma	RBC	Total Blood
Male	40–48	37–40	70–85
Female	37–46	22–27	59–73

SOURCE: After Opal Hepler, "Manual of Clinical Laboratory Methods," 4th ed. Used with permission of Charles C Thomas, Publisher, Springfield, Ill., 1954.

2. Draw blood for a dye-free control specimen, and, using the same needle and transferring syringes, inject dye into the patient in proportion to his body weight.
    After 1 h obtain a blood sample from the opposite arm, determine the percent of concentration of the dye in the plasma.

When radioactive chromate is used, at least three or four venipunctures must be made, depending upon the number of samples required after the radioactive-tagged cells are introduced. The department of nuclear medicine will instruct staff on individual preferences in regard to the time periods required to complete the evaluation.

EXAMINATION OF ERYTHROCYTES

General Considerations

The red blood cell is a remarkably constructed cell, well designed to accomplish its function, that of carrying oxygen from the lungs to the tissues and carbon dioxide from the tissues to the lungs for release from the body. These exchanges are possible because oxygen and carbon dioxide form a loose association with the hemoglobin molecule. Since hemoglobin is contained within the red blood cells, maximum utilization of the compound depends upon the surface area exposed to the gaseous atmospheres. This maximum

TABLE 3-2   CONDITIONS CAUSING CHANGES IN BLOOD VOLUME

Change	Portion changed	Condition
Increased blood volume	1. Cells increased	1. Polycythemia vera 2. Cardiac decomposition 3. Leukemia (WBC increased)
	2. Plasma increased	1. Cirrhosis of liver 2. Scurvy 3. Splenomegaly
	3. Both cells and plasma increased	1. Exposure to moderate heat 2. Hyperthyroidism
Decreased blood volume	1. Cells decreased	1. Chronic nephritis 2. Pernicious anemia
	2. Plasma decreased	1. Dehydration 2. Surgical shock 3. Addison's disease
	3. Both cells and plasma decreased	Hemorrhage

SOURCE: After Opal Hepler, "Manual of Clinical Laboratory Methods," 4th ed., 1954. Used with permission of Charles C Thomas, Publisher, Springfield, Ill.

efficiency is possible because of the shape of the red blood cell, which is a biconcave disk affording a large surface area for a relatively small cell. Another important and unique feature of the red blood cell is its flexibility. It is easily drawn out from its normal disk shape into a long narrow shape whenever necessary to ensure its passage through the fine capillaries, and it regains its normal shape in areas that will accommodate it.

DEVELOPMENT OF ERYTHROCYTES

From polychromatic megaloblast (the earliest form of erythrocyte) to reticulocyte (the erythrocyte that is released from the bone marrow into the peripheral circulation) requires about 7 days' development. An additional 4 days are required for the reticulocyte to reach complete maturity. Because an erythrocyte lacks a nucleus, it can carry out its intracellular metabolic activities for only a short time. This time equals the cell's life span. By means of tagging red blood cells with a radionuclide or by testing for transfused cells, it has been found that the usual life span of the red blood cell is about 120 days; i.e., about 120 days elapse between the time that the cell enters the peripheral circulation and the time that it becomes "worn out" and is removed from the circulation. When it is worn out, the erythrocyte is phagocytized by liver and spleen cells, which then break it down. Its hemoglobin content is further broken down into parts, and the process of rebuilding begins. Normally the simultaneous processes of removing old red blood cells and adding fresh ones proceed at the rate of about 50 ml/day.

TABLE 3-3   NORMAL VALUES FOR BLOOD COUNTS

Measure	Value
Hemoglobin	Men: 14.5–16.5 g/dl blood Women: 13.0–15.5 g/dl blood
Red blood cell count	Men: 4.8–5.5 million/mm^3 blood Women: 4.4–5.0 million/mm^3 blood
Hematrocrit	Men: 43–50 vol/dl Women: 40–45 vol/dl
Reticulocytes	0.5–1.5% of total RBC
White blood cell count	6,000–9,000/mm^3 blood
Differential count	Neutrophils: 60–70% of total WBC Eosinophils: 0–5% of total WBC Basophils: 0–3% of total WBC Lymphocytes*: 30–40% of total WBC Monocytes: 0–5% of total WBC

*Children normally may have a higher percentage of lymphocytes than adults. in red blood cell count and hemoglobin evaluation, their range of normal is about that of adult women.

TABLE 3-4   CHARACTERISTICS OF THE ERYTHROCYTE
IN HEALTH AND DISEASE

Term	Description of cell	Disease in which found
Normocyte	Normal RBC: 7–8 μm in diameter	
Microcyte	RBC smaller than normal	Secondary anemia
Macrocyte	RBC larger than normal	Primary anemia
Spherocyte	RBC uniformly round rather than biconcave	Hemoglobin C disease, thallassemia major
Anisocytosis	Variation in size of RBC	May be seen in any of the anemias
Poikilocytosis	Variation in shape of RBC	May be seen in any of the anemias
Basophilia	Bluish coloration of RBC	Chemical poisoning; may be seen in anemic conditions; when it occurs as dots (basophilic stippling), lead poisoning or thallassemia may be suspected
Normochromia	Normal buff-orange color of stained RBC	
Hypochromia	Pale-colored RBC due to low hemoglobin content	May be seen in any of the anemias
Target cell	Area of central pallor contains a "bull's eye"	Thalassemia, hemoglobin C disease, sickle cell anemia
Schistocyte	Fragmented cell	Severe anemias
Ovalocyte	Oval shape	Anemias; may also be familial
Elliptocyte	Longer than wide	Sickle cell anemia, familial
Siderocyte	Contains clumps of iron-bearing granules (Pappanheimer bodies)	Thalassemia; sickle cell anemia, postsplenectomy
Howell-Jolly body	Small, round, discrete blue nuclear remnant	Severe anemia, postsplenectomy
Heinz body	Coarse, violet-staining precipitate of hemoglobin	Anemias that are drug-induced or associated with unstable hemoglobin types

STRUCTURE OF ERYTHROCYTES

Mature red blood cells are the only nonnucleated cells of the body. In the erythrocytic series, the nucleus is present only in the immature cells. Only when there is a heavy demand on the hematopoietic system for replacement of red blood cells lost because of disease or severe hemorrhage do nucleated red blood cells appear in the peripheral circulation. In severe anemias, immature erythrocytes are released into the peripheral circulation. When these cells are present, they are noted in the results of the differential count (the study of the stained blood smear).

Estimation of Total Erythrocyte Count

Abbreviation: RBC
Normal range
Men: 4.8–5.5 million/mm^3
Women: 4.4–5.0 million/mm^3

METHOD

All total counts of blood cells are based on samples diluted so as to make counting feasible. Two methods are used in performing counts: visual and electronic. For the visual count, special pipets calibrated to measure the proper amounts of blood and diluent are used. Contained within the bulb of the pipet is a small bead which facilitates the mixture of the suspension of cells in diluent. For red cell counts, the standard dilution is 1:200. With the use of a microscope and a special glass slide called a *hemocytometer*, the number of cells in a prescribed area is counted, and calculations are made to account for the dilution and the depth of the counting chamber. The electronic counts are based on the fact that cells interrupt electric impulses when they pass through an electric field. These interruptions are translated onto a digital counter as the specified volume of cells per diluent passes through a calibrated aperture.

Hematocrit Test

Abbreviation: Hct
Normal range
  Men: 45–50 vol/dl
  Women: 40–45 vol/dl

EVALUATION

When defined literally, hematocrit means "to separate blood." This is precisely what is done in the hematocrit test, for the cellular elements are separated from the plasma by centrifugation. The results indicate the relative volumes of cells and plasma. This study of red blood cells is a valuable tool for the hematologist, for combining the findings of the red blood cell count, the hemoglobin concentration, and the hematocrit test will yield a great deal of information about the size, capacity, and number of cells. The results of the hematocrit test are expressed as cubic milliliters of packed cells per deciliter of blood or in volumes per deciliter of blood. It has become common practice to use the hematocrit reading as an indicator for the red blood cell count. When the hematocrit test is done on capillary blood (from a finger prick), the method is specified as "microhematocrit" because only a small amount of blood is used.

Reticulocyte Count

Abbreviation: retic
Normal range: 0.5–1.4% of total erythrocytes[1]

Reticulocytes are red blood cells that, when stained supravitally (in the living state), show fine networks of granular material. Red blood cells all have this *reticulum* present in the latter stages of development; this reticulum persists not more than 4 days after the cells have been released from the bone marrow into the peripheral circulation.

[1] This value is based on the assumption that the total erythrocyte count is within normal limits.

Reticulocyte counts are done in cases of suspected hemolytic or macrocytic anemias and as a routine check on persons working with radioactive material. An increase in the number of reticulocytes indicates that the formation of mature red blood cells is occurring more rapidly than normal. Thus a high count is seen when mature cells are lost or are prematurely destroyed. Examples include hemolytic anemias and destruction of mature cells by radioactive substances. In macrocytic anemias, on the other hand, red blood cell development is arrested before the reticulocyte stage is reached, so reticulocyte count is below normal. In the case of pernicious anemia (a macrocytic anemia), a sudden high count usually occurs after treatment is initiated. This indicates that the treatment is effective and red blood cell development is now making up lost time. In the same way, reticulocyte counts are useful for determining response to treatment for aplastic conditions.

Although it is not a common practice, it is extremely important to translate the relative reticulocyte count (as indicated by percent) into the absolute count when the total erythrocyte count is not within the normal range. The importance of this is seen in the following examples: If the erythrocyte count is 5.0 million and the reticulocyte count 1 percent, the absolute value is 5,000 reticulocytes ml^3, or normal. A reticulocyte count of 10 percent with 2.0 million erythrocytes 1 ml^3 would be the equivalent of 25 percent if the total count were 5.0 million. Conversely, an erythrocyte count of 7.0 million with 7 percent reticulocytes would correspond to 5 percent with a 5.0 million erythrocyte count. Since many of the cases in which reticulocyte counts are done involve lower-than-normal erythrocyte counts, the relative numbers of reticulocytes can be quite misleading in judging the patient's response to therapy, and it is imperative that absolute counts be used for this purpose.

METHOD

A drop of blood is mixed with a special dye and allowed to stand for a few minutes to complete the staining process. The blood is then spread in a film on cover slips or glass slides, and the number of reticulocytes counted among a total of 1,000 red blood cells is recorded. This result is then divided by 10 to obtain the percent of reticulocytes present. It is necessary to count this relatively high number of red blood cells in order to assure a good statistical sampling of the specimen.

Erythrocyte Fragility

Abbreviation: RBC frag
Normal range
   Beginning hemolysis: 0.44–0.42% saline solution
   Complete hemolysis: 0.34% saline solution

There is a normal rate of destruction of red blood cells, but when this rate increases perceptibly, anemia results. It is helpful to determine whether the increased rate of destruction is due in part to rupture of the red blood cells. In congenital hemolytic jaundice, for instance, the fragility of the red blood cells is increased; whereas in acquired hemolytic anemias the red blood cells show normal fragility. This is evidence that hemolysis in the latter instance is due to toxic hemolytic agents or to an immune type of hemolytic agent.

METHOD

A drop of blood is placed in each tube of a series containing decreasing amounts of saline concentrations. All the concentrations are hypotonic; i.e., the osmotic pressure exerted by the saline solution is less than that exerted from within the red blood cell. When the cell is easily ruptured, this difference in osmotic pressures facilitates the process. Normal cells are able to resist the lower osmotic pressures of hypotonic solutions until the saline concentration is lowered from 0.85% (concentration of physiologic saline solution) to about 0.44%.

Hemoglobin

Abbreviations: Hgb or HB

Normal range[1]
  Men: 14.5-16.0 g/dl blood
  Women: 13.0-15.5 g/dl blood

Hemoglobin is the respiratory pigment protein of mammals. Its respiratory function is evidenced by its ability to form a loose (i.e., easily reversed) chemical combination with oxygen and carbon dioxide. The molecule of hemoglobin is huge, being made up of 8,000 atoms (compare with the water molecule, which is composed of 3 atoms). It is a protein structure built of 600 amino acids of 19 different kinds.

The hemoglobin molecule is made up of two pairs of chains of amino acids, which form the globin portion, and of four prosthetic heme groups, each containing one atom of ferrous iron. By studies of molecular structure and electrophoretic patterns, about 200 types of hemoglobin have been identified. The types are distinguished by the substitution of one amino acid for another in the sequence of amino acids comprising the globin chains. Because hemoglobin is a protein, hemoglobin type is a genetically controlled characteristic. Hemoglobin types are designated by letter and/or by a proper noun, such as city or surname. Hemoglobin A is normal adult hemoglobin; hemoglobin F, fetal hemoglobin; hemoglobin S, that associated with sickle cell anemia. Abnormal hemoglobins are termed hemoglobinopathies. Hemoglobin F is normal during fetal life and during the first 4 months of postnatal life. It is present only in traces in the adult. It is, however, associated with some anemias due to hemoglobinopathy, most with particularly thalassemia, in which there is reduced production of one of the globin chains, usually the beta chain.

Another classification of hemoglobin is based on the ability of the heme portion of the hemoglobin molecule to form complexes. This classification is indicated below:

Oxyhemoglobin   Heme + oxygen

[1]The results are sometimes reported in percent, but this is an artificial term of reference because the value in grams per deciliter chosen to represent 100 percent may vary from place to place; similarly, the value in grams per deciliter chosen to represent 100 percent for men is different from that used for women.

Reduced hemoglobin	Heme without oxygen
Carboxyhemoglobin	Heme + carbon monoxide
Sulfhemoglobin	Heme + sulfur
Methemoglobin	Heme in which the ferrous ion is oxidized to the ferric state by some agent other than oxygen, e.g., by nitrites

Detection of these chemically different hemoglobins is by means of spectrosocpy.

METHODS OF DETERMINING AMOUNT OF HEMOGLOBIN

A number of methods have been devised in an attempt to find one that is both accurate and simple. In some of them, such as the Dare or Tallquist methods, both of which depend on matching a spot of blood from the patient with that of a standard, simplicity sacrifices accuracy. In the Sahli and Haden-Hausser methods, the hemoglobin is reduced to acid hematin by mixing the blood with a weak solution of hydrochloric acid, and the color is then matched to standards. This is done by inspection and is, therefore, subject to human error in discerning differences in color.

The method of choice is the cyanmethemoglobin method, which measures all forms of hemoglobin except sulfhemoglobin. With this method, the color intensity is measured in the photometer rather than by inspection, thus assuring accuracy.

ERYTHROCYTE INDEXES

The relationship between the number, size, and hemoglobin content of the erythrocytes is important in accurately describing anemias. The terms used in these descriptions refer to the hemoglobin content and the size of the cells. A rough index of these elements may be obtained from an inspection of the stained peripheral-blood smear and a description using the terms indicated on the following page.

Term	Definition
Normochromic	Normal color (i.e., normal hemoglobin content)
Hypochromic	Less than normal color
Normocytic	Normal size of cells
Microcytic	Smaller than normal size
Macrocytic	Larger than normal size

Note that the term "hyperchromic" is not used. To put it in a homely phrase, a bucket can only hold so much water—a red blood cell, being a container, can hold only a given amount of hemoglobin. Cells which appear to be much darker than normal, owe their darkness to shape (spherocytosis) rather than to hemoglobin content. Precise measures of size and hemoglobin content are obtained by combining determinations of hemoglobin, erythrocyte count, and hematocrit. Normal values for the various erythrocyte indexes are given in Table 3-5.

Anemias

The body has a remarkably economical system for synthesizing hemoglobin. The life span of the red blood cell is about 120 days. The materials that make up the hemoglobin of the cells is recycled. It will be noted that the iron is stored for reuse. The turnover of iron in the body, i.e., excretion and then absorption of fresh supplies, is rather slow, assuring an adequate supply of this mineral under

TABLE 3-5   ERYTHROCYTE INDEXES

Index	Normal Value	Measurement made
Color index	0.90–1.0	Rough estimate of concentration of hemoglobin in cells
Mean corpuscular hemoglobin concentration	30–36 g/dl packed RBC	Average hemoglobin content per dl packed RBCs
Mean corpuscular hemoglobin	29–32 μg^{-6}	Average amount of hemoglobin per cell
Mean corpuscular volume	82–96 μm^3	Average size of individual cell

normal circumstances. Disruption of iron utilization or exhaustion of iron supply will be reflected in studies of total serum iron. When iron is not being utilized optimally, there will be an increase in residual iron. Of course, if the problem is lack of absorption of ingested iron, the residual iron will not rise or keep pace with demands. Obviously, any influence external to the hematopoietic system which alters this rate will affect the total red blood cell count and the level of hemoglobin. Thus, as is seen in polycythemia vera, the replacement of red blood cells proceeds at a rate faster than that at which old cells are removed, and a very high red blood cell count results. When the replacement apparatus is impaired, the red blood cell count falls and the hemoglobin level is reduced, producing anemia.

Anemia is *never* a diagnosis, but rather a laboratory finding, just as headache is a symptom and hepatomegaly a physical finding. Anemia may be dignified by being called a secondary diagnosis, but one must not stop there, or the patient's health and/or life may be jeopardized. Therapy directed toward treating the red blood cell count may only mask the condition causing the low count. To avoid this, a primary diagnosis must be established. For example, the earliest finding of gastrointestinal cancer may be a slight anemia, and the blood findings may be "cured" by transfusions, but the cancer grows larger. The cure of this anemia comes only through diligent efforts leading to the real diagnosis, not of anemia, but of cancer, and the subsequent application of appropriate treatment. Another example of the principle involved in establishing diagnosis is the statement that normocytic normochromic anemia is a *finding* of malnutrition; malnutrition is the *diagnosis.* There is no laboratory test that takes the place of a careful history and complete physical examination, especially when dealing with a symptom of anemia. The function of the laboratory tests is to supplement the information gained from the history and physical examination.

There are a number of systems of classification of anemias, depending on the focus for the various categories. The simplest separates anemias into primary (associated with defective hematopoiesis) and secondary (associated with extrahematopoietic conditions). Table 3-6 shows examples of the relationships between underlying

TABLE 3-6 EXAMPLES OF TYPES OF ANEMIAS

Cause	Predominant RBC morphology	Examples of conditions in which seen
Impairment of RBC maturation due to deficiency of vitam B_{12} or folic acid	Macrocytes Poikilocytes Anisochromic	Pernicious anemia, sprue, postgastrectomy, celiac disease
Acute blood loss	Normocytic Normochromic	Trauma, hemophilic hemorrhage, acute hemorrhage associated with other disease such as malignancy
Intravascular hemolysis corpuscular defect	Morphologic changes vary; predominant types typical of specific RBC defect	Corpuscular defects, e.g., membrane, metabolic abnormality. May be spherocytosis, RBC enzyme defects, elliptocytosis
Extracorpuscular agents	Normochromic Normocytic	Drug-sensitive RBC, vegetable or animal poisons, malaria, bacteria (*Clostridium welchii, Vibrio cholerae*), incompatible transfusion, hemolytic autoimmune antibodies
Iron deficiency	Microcytes Hypochromic	Low dietary intake, chronic diarrhea, postgastrectomy, sprue, closely spaced pregnancies, high growth requirements
Impaired formation	Microcytes	Chronic inflammatory diseases

TABLE 3-6   EXAMPLES OF TYPES OF ANEMIAS (continued)

Cause	Predominant RBC Morphology	Examples of conditions in which seen
Chronic blood loss	Microcytes Hypochromic	"Silent" alimentary or genitourinary-tract bleeding, malignancies
Hemoglobinopathies	Morphology varies, with predominant forms being those associated with the particular hemoglobinopathy (e.g., target cells, sickle cells)	Sickle cell anemia, thalassemia, hemoglobin C disease, heterozygous hemoglobinopathy (e.g., sickle/C), paroxysmal nocturnal hemoglobinuria
Impaired production	Anisocytosis may be shown, but primarily normocytic, normochromic	Marrow suppression due to antimetabolites, intentional or accidental radiation, poisonous chemicals
	Normocytic to microcytic with hypochromasia	Chronic renal disease, collagen disease, extramedullary malignancy, chronic infection
Malignant infiltration of the bone marrow	Anisocytosis Poikilocytosis Anisochromia	Leukemias, myeloma, malignancies metastatic to the bone

cause, types of morphology seen, and some examples of diseases associated with each. This table is neither fully detailed nor comprehensive. It is intended only to show examples.

Erythrocyte Sedimentation Rate

Abbreviation: sed rate or ESR
Normal ranges

Method	Men, mm/h	Women, mm/h
Cutler	0–8	0–10
Wintrobe	0–6.5	0–15
Westergren	0–15	0–20

EVALUATION

The rapidity with which the red blood cells settle out of the un-clotted blood in 1 h constitutes the sedimentation rate.[1] This rate of fall of the red blood cells has been found to depend, to some degree, on alterations of the blood proteins. These alterations render the red blood cells more likely to stack up together like coins (rouleau formation), which increases the rate of fall due to the mere weight of the cell aggregates. The different methods listed above have different normal ranges because the bore and length of the tube used in each method differs. These factors influence the rate of fall markedly, as can be seen by comparison of the ranges.

This test is entirely nonspecific. To some hematologists, it is an unreliable test because it is so frequently inconclusive and at variance with clinical findings. It is affected by physiologic factors as well as by disease. It has been said of the sedimentation rate that it "doesn't tell where the fire is, but does tell how hot it is." In general, it is used as a rough index of the progress of an inflammatory disease, particularly rheumatoid arthritis, rheumatic fever, and respiratory infections. However, for these diseases other tests which are more sensitive and specific are available, and the sedimentation rate is used less frequently, although it remains an old standby. Sedimentation-rate results are viewed subjectively and must be interpreted in the light of the careful clinical evaluations.

[1] This is not to be confused with urinary sediment studies—a common misunderstanding.

EXAMINATION OF LEUKOCYTES

Abbreviation: WBC
Normal range: total WBC 6,000–9,000/mm³

General Considerations

The term *leukocyte* is derived from the appearance of the concentrated white blood cells that lie atop the packed red blood cells when unclotted blood is centrifuged. The term *buffy coat* refers to this layer of cells specifically and may be mentioned in the report of the hematocrit test.

Leukocytes are classified in two major groups, or series: *polymorphonuclear* and *mononuclear*. In the former, as the name indicates, the nucleus is many-shaped or has a tendency to develop into lobular shapes. In addition, the cells in this series have granules

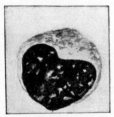 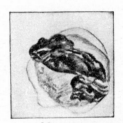

Lymphocyte   Monocyte

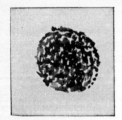 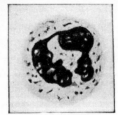 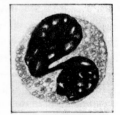

Basophil   Neutrophil   Eosinophil

FIG. 3-2 Normal mature leukocytes. *(Redrawn from S.E. Miller, "Textbook of Clinical Pathology," 4th ed., The Williams & Wilkins Company, Baltimore, 1952, by permission of the publisher.)*

in the cytoplasm which further distinguish them one from another. Cells with granules that are neutral in staining reaction are *neutrophils*; cells with granules that are acidic in staining reaction are *eosinophils*; cells with granules that are basic in staining reaction are *basophils*. All three types arise from bone marrow and are therefore also classified as *myelogenous* cells.

The outline below shows the characteristics, functions, and common names of the three groups of polymorphonuclear cells. The cell names listed under neutrophil are those used to describe the cell as it progresses to maturity, and they may be applied to the other polymorphonuclear granulocytes as well.

Polymorphonuclear Granulocytes (Fig. 3-2)

1. Neutrophils (poly or seg); function: phagocytosis
   a. Myeloblasts: very immature form seen in bone marrow
   b. Promyelocytes: immature form seen in peripheral circulation in myelogenous leukemias
   c. Metamyelocytes: fairly young form, sometimes called "juvenile," which may be seen in the peripheral blood in myelogenous leukemia or in severe infection with markedly elevated WBC
   d. "Bands"[1] : early mature form, seen in greater numbers in peripheral blood when WBC count is elevated
   e. "Segmenters"[2] : mature cells, normally comprising the majority of neutrophils
2. Eosinophils (eo); function: not completely determined, but they play some role in allergic conditions, possibly as an antihistamine
3. Basophils (baso); function: not completely determined, but they may play some role in preventing coagulation in inflamed areas, keeping the area fluid, and preventing stasis

---

[1] This name describes the shape of the nucleus, which is somewhat sausage-shaped, with no indentation.

[2] This name also describes the shape of the nucleus: in this cell, the sausage-shaped nucleus is pinched off into lobes, or segments, with a filament connecting the lobes. There are usually three to five lobes.

In the mononuclear series are *lymphocytes, monocytes,* and *plasmocytes.* These cells originate primarily in the lymphoid tissue, although plasmocytes grow around blood vessels and are commonly seen in aggregates in these areas. The functions of lymphocytes are to wall off chronic infections and to produce antibodies. Monocytes, too, are involved in these processes, and they also function as phagocytes, although not as actively as do neutrophils. The plasmocytes produce antibodies and other proteins. They are not ordinarily seen in the peripheral circulation. The outline below shows the development and common names of the mononuclear series.

Mononuclear Cells (Fig. 3-2)

1. Lymphocytes (lymph); function: walling off chronic infections, producing antibodies
   a. Prolymphocytes: immature cells seen in peripheral blood in acute lymphocytic leukemias
   b. Lymphoblasts: immature cells seen in peripheral blood in lymphocytic leukemias
   c. Atypical lymphocytes: characteristic cells seen in infectious mononucleosis
2. Monocytes (mono); function: some phagocytosis
   a. Promonocytes: immature cells seen in peripheral blood in monocytic leukemia
   b. Monoblasts: immature cells not seen in the peripheral blood except in monocytic leukemia
3. Plasmocytes; function: producing antibodies and some globulin; fairly frequently seen in the peripheral blood in multiple myeloma

Estimation of Total Leukocyte Count

As with the total red blood cell count, the blood is diluted in a special pipet to facilitate counting and to dissolve the red blood cells. The usual diluent is 1% hydrochloric acid. The hemocytometer is used, and a given area is counted; then calculations are made for dilution factor (1:20) and depth of counting chamber, and the results are given as number of white blood cells per cubic millimeter. Blood is obtained by finger prick or venipuncture. As is the case in erythrocyte counts, the electronic cell counter is used routinely.

Differential Count

Abbreviation: diff
Normal ranges:
Adults

Cell	% of total white count
Neutrophils	60–70
Eosinophils	0–5
Basophils	0–3
Lymphocytes	30–40
Monocytes	0–5

Children: usually show a higher percentage of lymphocytes
Source of blood: finger prick or venipuncture

EVALUATION

An important part of the white blood cell count is the differential count, so called because it is a tabulation of the relative numbers of the various types of white blood cells that constitute the total count. It yields valuable information and should never be omitted from the count, for information not apparent in the total count could very well be demonstrated in the morphology and/or distribution of the various cells. It is important in judging the red blood cells as well, because it shows their morphology and provides a rough estimate of their hemoglobin content. Both morphology and a rough estimate of the number of platelets provide additional important information for evaluating various hematologic problems.

RELATIVE AND ABSOLUTE VALUES

As is the case of any measurement, such as percent, which is based on relative quantities, it is important to keep in mind the *absolute* values in differential counts, in terms of the number of cells per cubic millimeter. When one uses only the percentage of cells present, as indicated in the routine differential count, one can be misled. For example, a report of 50 percent lymphocytes might be taken to mean a lymphocytosis if it is considered only at face value. However, when the total leukocyte count is considered, the interpretation can be altered. If, in the case of 50 percent lymphocytes, the total leukocyte count is $2,500/mm^3$, the absolute count would fall within the normal range (see Table 3-7). Thus, one would not investigate further on the false assumption that lymphocytosis existed, but would recognize that a relative lymphocytosis with leukopenia (indicated by the low total count) is, in reality, a neutropenia. The investigation then would be focused on the existent condition which would cause a lowering of the number of neutrophils in the blood.

Another example of the use to be made of absolute values is seen in the case of a patient whose total leukocyte count was 1,800, with 11 percent eosinophils. Eosinophilia is known to occur in

TABLE 3-7   COMPARISON OF RELATIVE AND ABSOLUTE VALUES
IN ADULT DIFFERENTIAL COUNTS

Cells	Average* (absolute)	Range* (absolute)	% (relative)
Total leukocytes	7,000	5,000–10,000	100
Total neutrophils	4,300	3,000–7,000	60–70
Segmenters	4,300	3,000–5,800	54–65
Young forms	300	150–400	3–5
Lymphocytes	2,100	1,500–3,000	20–30
Monocytes	375	285–500	2–6
Eosinophils	200	50–400	1–4
Basophils	25	0–50	0–1

*Figures are in terms of number of cells per cubic millimeter of whole blood.

some parasitic diseases, and a search for intestinal parasites was erroneously begun, because the relative value for eosinophils was misleading. When the absolute values were calculated, it was seen that the number of eosinophils present was well within normal range, and the search for parasites was abandoned. Table 3-7 shows a comparison between relative and absolute values in adult differential counts.

A term which may sometimes be met is *shift to the left*, indicating an increase in the younger forms of the neutrophils. This term is derived from the notation of the various young forms in tabular reports, the youngest forms being in the extreme-left column and the mature neutrophils at the extreme right. Shifts to the left may be due to regenerative or degenerative influences. A regenerative shift indicates release of the younger forms from the bone marrow in response to a heavy demand for neutrophils, such as is seen in acute infections. A degenerative shift to the left indicates a block in the maturation process, with the release of immature cells rather than mature cells.

Special Stains

A variety of cellular inclusions are identified in the proper study of the stained blood smear. In some instances, special stains are required to visualize the inclusions in leukocytes or to identify chemical components.

The *leukocyte alkaline phosphatase stain (LAP)* is used to distinguish between leukemoid reactions and leukemia. Leukemoid reactions are sometimes seen in severe infections, in which myelocytes and metamyelocytes (immature granulocytes) are seen in the peripheral blood in response to the infection. LAP is present in diffuse, heavy granules in the granulocytic cells of leukemoid reactions and in those of patients with polycythemia vera.

The *leukocyte peroxidase stain* is used to distinguish between the blast cells of granulocytic and mononuclear series and assists in distinguishing between acute myelocytic leukemia and acute lymphocytic leukemia. The granulocytic series of cells contain scattered blue granules in the cytoplasm (particularly in the neutrophils) when stained for peroxidase.

The *nitroblue tetrazolium (NBT)* test is used primarily to assist in distinguishing viral infections (which give a negative result) from bacterial and fungal infections and noninfectious febrile diseases (the latter three give positive results). It is considered by some to be useful in monitoring patients who are subject to high risk of infection, such as those under immunosuppressive regimens. Colorless nitroblue tetrazolium is reduced to a dense blue-black precipitate of formazon, probably by enzymes associated with phagocytosis.

TABLE 3-8   LEUKOCYTE MORPHOLOGY AND INCLUSIONS

Morphology/inclusion	Description
Doehle body	Small, blue aggregate in cytoplasm of neutrophils; remnant of cytoplasmic RNA; associated with May-Hegglin anomaly and may be seen in infectious diseases
Reilly bodies (Adler-Reilly anomaly)	Scattered, coarse, blue-staining granules primarily in neutrophils; associated with mucopolysaccharidosis (gargoylism)
Toxic granulation	Dark-staining, scattered granules in neutrophil cytoplasm; seen in severe infections or toxic states
Pelger-Huet Anomaly	Marked predominance of band forms of the granulocytes in the absence of infection; familial and nonpathologic, but must be distinguished from "shift to the left" with immature neutrophils as seen in severe infections
Auer body	Splinter-shaped azurophilic body in the cytoplasm of granulocytes, particularly neutrophilic series; associated with acute myelocytic leukemia and may also be seen in acute monocytic leukemia

LUPUS ERYTHEMATOSUS CELLS

Abbreviation: LE prep
Normal range: no LE cells present
Unit of measure: number of LE cells/100 leukocytes or "none seen"

The LE cell is a characteristic cell seen in approximately 60 percent of cases of lupus erythematosus (LE). It is a phagocytic polymorphonuclear cell that has ingested altered nuclear material. Not all cases of LE will demonstrate the cell, and those that do show it may not do so consistently. Consequently, repeated examinations may be necessary before the diagnosis of LE can be ruled out by laboratory methods. The antinuclear antibody test may also be used in the diagnosis of lupus erythematosus.

EXAMINATION OF THROMBOCYTES

Alternate name: platelets
Normal range: 200,000–350,000/mm^3

The term *thrombocyte* means, literally, "clot cell." An important factor in blood coagulation, thrombocytes (more commonly called *platelets*) are small azure-colored bodies which, upon disintegration and clumping, contribute to the coagulation mechanism. Their adhesive quality makes them clump readily and stick to an injured or rough surface. Because of their retraction properties, they help to form, with fibrin, a dense network for the clot. Serotonin, which aids in vasoconstriction, is adsorbed on platelets. When platelets disintegrate, a substance very similar to thromboplastin (sometimes called "incomplete thromboplastin") is released. It interacts with other precursors of coagulation elements, forming complete thromboplastin, which then enters the coagulation mechanism.

While a normal number of platelets must be present to provide optimal coagulability for the blood, there are also qualitative aspects which can be involved, such as the amount of serotonin, the quality of thromboplastin, or the degree of adhesiveness. Platelet size can also be a factor in their function. Hence, it is important to describe the morphology of platelets as seen on the differential smear, as well as the actual numbers present.

Platelet deficiencies may be due to quantitative or qualitative types. In quantitative deficiencies, there is obviously a low total platelet count, as indicated by the term "thrombocytopenia." The prevailing opinion on the causes of thrombocytopenia is that they are due to an antibody-antigen reaction induced by a drug or toxic episode or to some autogenous mechanism. Of course, any drug which suppresses bone-marrow activity will have an effect on platelet production, since the marrow is the site of their formation. When adequate numbers of platelets are present, but their function is impaired, the condition is known as thromboasthenia.

HEMOSTASIS

Studies in Hemostasis

The phenomenon of blood coagulation has been the subject of observation and investigation since antiquity. As is to be expected, elucidation of the mechanisms involved in coagulation awaited the development of precise knowledge and instrumentation. The broader term *hemostasis* is preferred by modern investigators, since it is recognized that there is more involved than the coagulation processes per se; for instance, vasoconstriction is a particularly important factor.

Aristotle and Hippocrates explained coagulation as being due to lowering temperatures, and they were followed by others who extended this explanation by noting the effects of cessation of blood flow. Beginning in the mid-eighteenth century with the work of Hewson (1772), more sophisticated theories were developed, evolving into the modern concepts, which owe a great deal to the work of Morawitz (1905). It is now recognized that coagulation occurs in three steps:

Stage 1:   Formation of thromboplastic activity
Stage 2:   Conversion of prothrombin to thrombin
Stage 3:   Conversion of fibrinogen to fibrin

These processes do not occur as isolated events but, accompanied by other mechanisms which enhance and maintain hemostasis, are dynamic processes which are both sequential and simultaneous.

Contributing to the first stage are platelets, calcium, and thromboplastin precursors (factors VIII, IX, X, and XI). With the generation of thromboplastin, the stage is set for the second act: the thromboplastin serves as a catalyst upon prothrombin and accessory factors (factors V, VII, and VIII) to produce thrombin. The thrombin then acts upon fibrinogen to produce fibrin, the polymerized network of the clot, which traps erythrocytes. Platelets then play their second role, clot retraction, which shrinks the clot mass into a smaller volume and squeezes out the serum.

Table 3-9 lists the known coagulation factors and when and by whom they were discovered. To avoid the confusion which is inevitable when many synonyms are given, the International Committee for the Standardization of the Nomenclature of Blood Clotting Factors established the use of Roman numerals with the corresponding preferred name. Some of the names given to factors are derived from the surnames of the patients involved in their isolation (e.g., the Christmas and Hageman factors).

Clinical and Laboratory Studies
In Hemorrhagic Disorders

GENERAL CONSIDERATIONS

The most important preliminary to any laboratory studies in hemorrhagic disorders is a careful clinical history, for this can provide clues unobtainable in any other way and cause subsequent investigation to be intelligently focused upon a proper choice of tests. It is important to remember that many of the regularly used tests are limited by insensitivity to mild or moderate forms of disease which, when the patient is subjected to even so-called minor surgery, can cause serious hemorrhage. This history obtained must include points related to family history of bleeding tendencies. Other essential information to be obtained includes:

TABLE 3-9   COAGULATION FACTORS

Factor	Name or substance	Source, characteristics, function
I	Fibrinogen (1856, Virchow)	Produced in the liver. Protein present in plasma at an average level of 300 mg/dl. When acted upon by thrombin, forms firbrin.
II	Prothrombin (1860, Schmidt)	Produced in the liver, with vitamin K an essential part. Glycoprotein present in plasma; measured according to its activity. When acted upon by thromboplastin, forms thrombin.
III	Thromboplastin (1960, Schmidt)	Tissues and platelets (incomplete); plasma (complete). Incomplete forms require factors V, VII, X. Complete form is a product of interaction between factors VIII, IX, XI and platelets. Acts upon prothrombin to form thrombin.
IV	Calcium (1875, Hammersten)	Obtained from diet. Present in serum at levels of 4.8–5.2 meq/liter. Is an inorganic ion required in all stages of coagulation as an activator of enzyme activity.
V	Labile factor (1943, Owren)	Derived from plasma globulin. Found in normal plasma; used up in the clotting process; deteriorates rapidly at room temperature. Accelerates conversion of prothrombin to thrombin.
VI	Unassigned	In early studies, was thought to be the active form of factor V.
VII	Stable factor (1948, Owren and Bollman)	Produced in the liver. Not consumed in clotting, therefore present in normal serum. Stable to heat and storage. Accelerates the conversion of prothrombin to thrombin.

TABLE 3-9 (continued)

Factor	Name or substance	Source, characteristics, function
VIII	Antihemophiliac globulin (1936, Patek and Stetson)	Derived from plasma globulin. Completely consumed in clotting. Unstable at room temperature. Essential to the formation of thromboplastin and conversion of prothrombin to thrombin.
IX	Plasma thromboplastin component (Christmas factor) (1952, Aggeler)	Produced in the liver. Not consumed during clotting. Influences amount of thromboplastin generated.
X	Stuart-Prower factor (1952)	Probably produced in the liver, with vitamin K essential. Present in normal plasma and serum. Stable at room temperature. Similar to factor VII. Essential to generation of thromboplastin and activity of prothrombin.
XI	Plasma thromboplastin antecedent (1953, Rosenthal)	Site of synthesis unknown. Present in normal plasma and serum. Stable. Essential to formation of plasma, thromboplastin.
XII	Hageman factor (1955, Ratnoff)	Site of synthesis unknown. Relatively stable. Activated on contact with glass. Physiologic role not completely known.
XIII	Fibrin stabilizing factor (1962, Lorand and Dickeman)	Site of synthesis not known. High levels in plasma. Deficiency associated with mild bleeding tendency; poor wound healing. Maintains firm clot after formation.

1. The patient's age at the time symptoms of bleeding tendency were first noticed. During infancy, bleeding is uncommon except at circumcision or in vitamin K deficiency.

2. Any episodes of spontaneous bleeding—large bruises or hematuria. Multiple bruises (2 to 3 cm) are commonly seen in women and children but are not of great significance.
3. Type and degree of bleeding after dental extraction, minor surgery, or accidents.

Since hemostasis involves capillary function as well as the coagulation process, differentiation must be made by evaluation of the history and by interpretation of the test that discriminate between the two. Table 3-10 provides a comparison between capillary and coagulation defects in relation to specific conditions. Alertness in observing and reporting these effects may well contribute significantly to diagnosis of hemorrhagic tendencies.

The several tests for state of hemostasis are described in the following pages.

BLEEDING TIME

Abbreviation: bl time
Normal range: 3–6 min (Ivy method)

Although this test is notoriously abused in the way in which it is performed, it can provide clues as to the functional capacity of platelets and of vasoconstriction. It is important that the Ivy method be used, since it requires procedures which better control the variables inherent in the test. A puncture wound 2.5 mm deep is made on the volar surface of the forearm after a blood-pressure cuff has been placed on the arm and the pressure maintained at 40 mm Hg. The blood produced from the wound is carefully blotted at half-minute intervals until bleeding ceases. Bleeding time is prolonged in patients with vascular abnormalities, thrombocytopenia, and thromboasthenia. It is frequently necessary to repeat the test, since it is subject to variables which can readily alter results.

CLOT RETRACTION

Normally, retraction of the clot is observed within 2 h and is complete within 24 h.

TABLE 3-10   COMPARISON OF CAPILLARY AND
COAGULATION DEFECTS

Check list	Effect of coagulation defect	Effect of capillary defect
Bleeding from *small* superficial cuts	Often no excessive bleeding	Bleeding often profuse
Time of onset of bleeding	Often delayed 1–3 h	Usually immediate
Effect of pressure on lesion	Bleeding begins again after pressure is released	Bleeding often stopped permanently
Most common sites in severely affected individuals	Joints, muscles, massive subcutaneous bruises; any form of internal hemorrhage is common	Gastrointestinal bleeding, epistaxis, menorrhagia; large bruises less common; joints, muscles rarely involved
Symptoms in mildly affected individuals	Large hematoma following injury; persistent and often dangerous bleeding after trauma	Epistaxis, menorrhagia; traumatic bleeding less dangerous than with clotting defects

As noted above, the time and degree of contraction of an undisturbed clot depends upon platelet function. In thrombocytopenia, the clot retracts slowly and incompletely. In thromboasthenia, there is reduced clot retraction, and the clot formed is characteristically soft.

RUMPLE-LEEDS TOURNIQUET TEST

Normal: no petechiae result

Formally, this test is done by placing a blood-pressure cuff on an arm with the pressure midway between systolic and diastolic levels. After a 5-min period, the number of petechiae appearing are counted. Informally, the formation of such petechiae may be observed incidental to having the tourniquet on the patient's arm during the collection of a blood specimen.

FIBRINOGEN LEVEL

Normal range: 200–300 mg/dl plasma

Fibrinogen is a globulin protein of plasma that is essential in the process of coagulation. Nutritional deficiency may be the cause of fibrinogen levels that are moderately below normal, but, on the whole, the fibrinogen level remains quite constant under ordinary circumstances. Severe liver disease may produce low fibrinogen levels, since this protein is synthesized in the liver. Congenital afibrinogenemia has been seen, but it is a rare disease. Hypofibrinogenemia is a coagulation defect that may result in severe hemorrhage. Acquired hypofibrinogenemia is far more common than congenital hypofibrinogenemia and is sometimes a complication of pregnancy. It is sometimes a factor in hemorrhage resulting from neoplastic states or following surgery.

COAGULATION TIME

Abbreviation: coag time
Normal range: 9–12 min (Lee-White method)

This is an in vitro test using venous blood; it involves every factor in the coagulation mechanism. Individual laboratory techniques may cause results to vary somewhat from those given in the texts, making it essential that one know the range of normal values for the particular laboratory. The capillary-tube method is of little or no value, and its use should be discouraged. The coagulation time should never be used as a screening test, since it is not sensitive enough to detect mild to moderate hemorrhagic tendencies.

PROTHROMBIN TIME

Abbreviation: pro time or PT
Normal range: 12–15 s

This test measures the activity of five different coagulation factors: prothrombin, fibrinogen, and factors V, VII, and X. The prothrombin time is determined by adding known quantities of thromboplastin and calcium ions to a specified volume of plasma and noting the length of time for coagulation to occur. Determination of the prothrombin time is essential in any study of the co-

agulation process and in establishing and maintaining anticoagulant therapy.

The prothrombin time is prolonged when (1) the level of fibrinogen is less than 100 mg/dl plasma, (2) heparin has been given,
(3) prothrombin activity is impaired, (4) there is deficiency in
factor V, VII, or X, or (5) antithrombin circulating anticoagulants
are present.

A major source of difficulty in understanding the results reported for prothrombin times has been the terms used in these reports. The safest method of reporting is to note both the patient's
and the control times. This is best, since the measurement is one of
activity rather than quantitation, and the time required for completion of clotting is related to activity as much as to the amounts of
the factors measured. The therapeutic range for prothrombin time,
in seconds, is about twice that of the normal control; e.g., 24 if the
control is 12 s.

A commonly used method of reporting is in terms of so-called
"percent of normal activity." Strict percent cannot be used, since
one must then assume a straight-line relationship between activity
and time. This does not obtain, as is seen in Fig. 3-3. The therapeutic range, as reported in percent of normal activity, is between
10 and 20 percent.

PROTHROMBIN CONSUMPTION

Normal range: almost complete consumption, as indicated by
                 clotting time of more than 20 s for serum

The purpose of this test is to determine the capacity to generate
thromboplastin. When a blood sample from a normal subject clots,
prothrombin is converted to thrombin. When this occurs, there is
little or no prothrombin remaining in the serum. However, if
there is a deficiency in the factors that form thromboplastin, only a
portion of the prothrombin will be converted. This will result in a
high residual amount of prothrombin in the serum and indicate the
need for further tests to determine the deficient factor or factors.
This test provides information regarding the first stage of co-

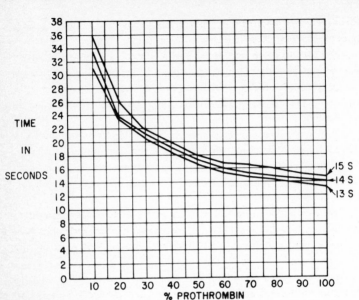

FIG. 3-3 Prothrombin-activity curves showing results for normal controls of 13, 14, and 15 s.

agulation; the results are abnormal when the first-stage factors (VII, IX, X and XI) are 10 percent or less or when platelets are reduced in number or efficiency.

THROMBOPLASTIN GENERATION

Abbreviation: TGT
Normal range: 12 s or less (100%)

It has been shown that blood can generate a powerful thromboplastin that is capable of clotting plasma in 8 to 12 s. Thromboplastin formed in this time is considered 100 percent. Factors necessary for production of thromboplastin are platelets, antihemophiliac factor (AHF), plasma thromboplastin component (PTC), plasma thromboplastin antecedent (PTA), and calcium ion. When an abnormal thromboplastin-generation test result is obtained, further tests are indicated to determine which factor is at fault. This is done by performing the thromboplastin-generation test using normal serum and substituting, one at a time, the patient's AHF, PTC, PTA, platelets, and serum. This test is useful in diagnosing hemophilias, in particular when making the distinction between classic hemophilia and Christmas disease.

PARTIAL THROMBOPLASTIN TIME

Abbreviation: PTT
Normal range: 39–53 s

This test is used as a screening test to discover deficiencies in all plasma factors other than VII. It is not applicable to cases involving platelet defects. As with the TGT, the precise factor deficiency must be found by substitution methods. The test is subject to a number of variables, and its reliability is directly influenced by careful technique carried out by an experienced laboratorian. Table 3-11 shows a comparison of diseases due to coagulation-factor deficiencies.

INTRAVASCULAR COAGULATION

Intravascular coagulation is a condition in which there is activation of the coagulation process internally, producing symptoms of bleeding which are similar to those of the coagulation-factor deficiencies. It may be local or disseminated. There is no simple explanation of the condition, since it is possible for one, or a combination of several, predisposing factors to precipitate the problem. Activation of the coagulation process in vivo may be due to introduction of tissue thromboplastic components due to disease or trauma, bacterial endotoxin, intravenous hemolysis, endothelial damage, stasis, or antigen-antibody complexes. The result of intravascular coagulation is depletion of component factors in coagulation to the degree that hemophilia is simulated.

The condition may be acute or chronic, with no history of prior bleeding tendency. The primary indicators of bleeding tendency are

TABLE 3-11   DISEASES DUE TO COAGULATION-FACTOR
DEFICIENCIES

Factor	Condition	Etiology	Treatment
I	Hypofibrinogenemia	Depletion of fibrinogen	Fibrinogen or plasma
II	Hypoprothrombin-emia	Liver function impaired, low levels of vitamin K_1, anticoagulant therapy	Symptomatic, plasma
III	Thrombocytopenia	Low platelets	Fresh blood or platelet con-centrate
IV	Hypocalcemia	Low calcium intake, low vitamin D intake, mul-tiple transfusions con-taining citrate	Intravenous calcium gluconate
V	Parahemophilia	Impaired liver function, congenital deficiency	Fresh blood or plasma
VII		Impaired liver function, anticoagulant therapy, congenital deficiency	Fresh blood or plasma
VIII	Hemophilia A (classic hemo-philia)	Congenital deficiency (sex-linked; occurs most frequently in males)	Fresh blood, frozen plasma, cryoprecipi-tate
VIII	von Willebrand's dis-ease	Low levels of factor VIII, vascular impairment, congenital deficiency	Fresh blood, frozen plasma, cryoprecipitate
IX	Hemophilia B	Congenital deficiency (sex-linked; occurs most fre-quently in males)	Fresh blood, frozen plasma, cryoprecipitate
	Christmas disease	Liver disease, vitamin K deficiency	Fresh blood, frozen plasma, cryoprecipitate
XI	Hemophilia C	Probably congenital (occurs in both sexes)	Fresh blood or plasma
XII		Congenital (important to distinguish this de-ficiency from that of the hemophilias)	Not needed

usually abnormal, such as low platelet count and prolonged prothrombin and partial thromboplastin times. Further investigation by
specific-factor analyses generally reveals low levels of fibrinogen and
of factors II, V, VIII, and XIII in acute disseminated intravascular
coagulation, but in chronic cases, these laboratory findings are not
necessarily characteristic. Diagnosis is usually difficult, requiring a
careful history and carefully controlled laboratory studies. Detection
of fibrin-fibrinogen degradation products (sometimes referred to as
fibrin split products) can also be useful in diagnosis of local or disseminated intravascular coagulation; again the detection calls for
carefully controlled laboratory studies. Blood specimens for these
studies should be drawn as soon as the diagnosis is suspected and
before blood transfusion is instituted.

ANTICOAGULANTS

Anticoagulant Therapy

HEPARIN

This compound is a mucopolysaccharide derived from liver. It
occurs naturally in man and in other animals. Its anticoagulative
property is caused by the inhibition of the conversion of prothrombin into thrombin, probably by inactivation of enzyme
activity.

The principal advantages of heparin therapy are its rapid action
and the ease with which it may be neutralized by intravenous
administration of protamine sulfate. Its effects are measured by the
whole-blood coagulation time, although it can also prolong the prothrombin time. Therapeutic levels are achieved when the coagulation
time is prolonged to about twice the normal value.

COUMARIN AND INDANDIONE DERIVATIVES

These compounds affect prothrombin and factors V and VII. In
contrast to heparin, the effects of these drugs are not noticeable for
12 to 36 h. There is a cumulative effect characteristic of therapy

with these drugs, so that maximal effect may not be noted for a period of 1 to 2 days. Dosage must be regulated, initially, on the basis of daily prothrombin-time tests, and thus standing orders for anticoagulant therapy should not be permitted.

Increased sensitivity to anticoagulant drugs has been noted in patients (1) with liver disease or hepatic congestion, (2) whose general nutrition is poor, (3) who are receiving large doses of aspirin, (4) who are receiving broad-spectrum antibiotics. The explanations of these sensitivities are quite logical. Since the liver is the site of synthesis of the coagulation factors involved, impairment of its function can decrease normal levels. Aspirin in large quantities is known to depress coagulation. Broad-spectrum antibiotics depress the normal bacterial flora of the intestinal tract, and since these organisms are important in the production of vitamin K (a component of prothrombin and factor VII), any diminution of this vitamin affects coagulation.

Any evidence of spontaneous bleeding from the mucous membranes or urinary tract should be brought to the attention of the physician at once. When major bleeding occurs during anticoagulant therapy with these drugs, blood transfusions and administration of vitamin K are indicated.

Anticoagulants Used in the Laboratory

In addition to understanding the application of anticoagulants in therapy, it is valuable to review the mechanisms of anticoagulants used in preparation of blood specimens for laboratory purposes.

HEPARIN

The effect of heparin, unlike those of the other compounds used as anticoagulants in the laboratory, is not permanent. It is not toxic, and therefore it is useful in transfusion therapy when multiple units of blood must be used; e.g., in open-heart surgery.

OXALATES

These are simple salts of oxalic acid—sodium, potassium, or ammonium oxalate. The principle of anticoagulation is based on the fact that oxalate precipitates calcium ions as calcium oxalate. These anticoagulants are used extensively in chemical determinations on blood. When ammonium oxalate is used, determinations for urea and nonprotein nitrogen may not be done, since these determinations involve testing for nitrogen levels. The nitrogen content of ammonia, therefore, would give erroneous results. *Oxalates are toxic.*

SEQUESTRENE

Sequestrene is ethylenediaminetetraacetic acid (EDTA). It holds calcium ions in nonionizable form by chelation. It is an extremely useful anticoagulant, since, unlike the oxalates, EDTA does not readily distort cell structure. It is nontoxic.

TRISODIUM CITRATE

Citrate holds calcium ions in nonionizable form, thus neutralizing their effectiveness. It is important in blood transfusions, being the principal anticoagulant used for this purpose. It is important also in studies involving plasma assays for coagulation factors, since it does not have deleterious effects on these factors as does oxalate.

TABLE 3-12   HEMATOLOGIC TEST RESULTS SEEN
IN THE MORE COMMON DISEASES

Test	Condition	Test results
Red blood cell count	1. Anemia	1. Less than 4.0 million; type of anemia determined in conjunction with other studies and clinical findings
	2. Polycythemia vera	2. More than 5.5 million
	3. Hemoconcentration	3. More than 5.5 million
White blood cell count and differential	1. Acute infections, such as a. Appendicitis	1. More than 10,000 a. Usually between 10,000 and 20,000, with moderate number of band forms
	b. Pneumonia (bacterial type)	b. May be very high, up to 30,000 or more, with many band forms
	c. Gastroenteritis	c. Higher than 20,000; may have moderate number of band forms
	2. Leukemia	2. May be extremely high (up to 200,000); many immature cells of the specific type of the leukemia; in chronic leukemias, fewer immature forms are seen
	3. Leukemoid reaction	3. Because of elevated WBC with immature forms, this response to an infection may be confused with leukemia
	4. Leukopenia a. Aleukemic leukemia	4. Less than 5,000 a. Immature forms are seen
	b. Aplastic bone marrow	b. Usually normal differential
	c. Some virus infections	c. Relative lymphocytosis
	d. Pancytopenia	d. Usually normal differential
	5. Infectious mononucleosis	5. May show either leukopenia or leukocytosis; many atypical lymphocytes are seen

TABLE 3-12   (continued)

Test	Condition	Test results
Hemoglobin	1. Anemia	1. Less than 12 g/dl
	2. Polycythemia vera	2. More than 16.5 g/dl
	3. Hemoconcentration	3. More than 16 g/dl
	4. Leukemia	4. Usually less than 10 g/dl
Reticulocyte count	1. Pernicious anemia	1. Less than 0.5% before treatment; marked increase after treatment
	2. Hemolytic anemia	2. More than 1.5%
	3. Aplastic anemia	3. Less than 0.5%
Platelet count	1. Thrombocytopenia	1. Less than 100,000
	2. Toxic effect on bone marrow (chemical or medicinal)	2. Less than 100,000
	3. Pancytopenia	3. Less than 100,000
Sedimentation rate	Acute inflammatory processes	More than 10 mm fall/h
Coagulation time	1. Thrombocytopenia	All longer than 12 min
	2. Hypofibrinogenemia	
	3. Impairment of one of coagulation factors	
	4. Anticoagulant therapy	
Prothrombin time	1. Hypoprothrombinemia	All more than 16 s
	2. Anticoagulant therapy (Dicumarol)	
	3. Severe liver diseases	
Thrombo-plastin-generation time	Impairment of AHF, PTC, PTA, or platelets	More than 12 s
Fibrinogen level	1. Severe liver disease	All less than 200 mg/dl plasma
	2. Afibrinogenemia	
	3. Hypofibrinogenemia	

REFERENCES

Davidson, Israel, and John B. Henry (eds.): "Todd-Sanford Clinical Diagnosis by Laboratory Methods," 15th ed., Saunders, Philadelphia, 1974.

Diggs, L. W., et al.: "The Morphology of Human Blood Cells," Saunders, Philadelphia, 1956.

Leitner, Stefan J.: "Bone Marrow Biopsy: Hematology in the Light of the Sternal Puncture," 2d ed., Grune & Stratton, New York, 1949.

Miale, John B.: "Laboratory Medicine—Hematology," 4th ed., Mosby, St. Louis, 1972.

Sirridge, Marjorie S.: "Laboratory Evaluation of Hemostasis," 2d ed., Lea & Febiger, 1974.

Williams, W. J. (ed.): "Hematology," McGraw-Hill, New York, 1972.

Wintrobe, Maxwell M.: "Clinical Hematology," 7th ed., Lea & Febiger, Philadelphia, 1972.

FOUR

BIOCHEMICAL EXAMINATIONS

Biochemical examinations impose some necessary restrictions upon the patient which she may feel are unreasonable. If she were not ill or facing the possibility of illness, it would probably be easier for her to deal with these restrictions. The majority of biochemical tests are done on blood samples drawn by venipuncture. This is one part of the procedure that can be simply explained, as noted in Chap. 3. Care must be taken to be sure the patient understands the reasons for the preparation for biochemical tests and the exact elements involved in procedures that require her intelligent cooperation. The results will be a better attitude on the part of the patient and, inevitably, more accurate tests. Put in dollars and cents, this means the patient gets more for her money.

GENERAL CONSIDERATIONS

In biochemical examinations, important considerations for nurses are (1) how to read and interpret the physician's orders, (2) how to help prepare the patient for the tests, and (3) how to read the test reports.

In addition to these considerations (which are rather detached from the patient), other advantages result when the nurse understands these examinations—advantages that enhance his ability in his unique position as link between the patient and her treatment and between the patient and the technologist. He is better able to plan his own activities in conjunction with those of the laboratory. Each of these factors result in better overall patient care.

Many laboratories make it a general rule to collect blood specimens for chemical work when the patient is in the postabsorptive state, i.e., has not eaten for at least 10 h. It is presumed easier to collect *all* specimens when the patient is in the fasting state than to have the nurse remember which tests are inaccurate if the specimen is not collected during fasting. It also provides a better base line for any particular patient when comparing repeated tests. An additional consideration is that it aids the laboratory a great deal in organizing the day's work if all specimens are collected the first thing in the morning. This general rule does not, of course, apply to emergency situations.

BLOOD-CHEMISTRY SCREENING TESTS

With the increasing attention being given to preventive medicine and the concomitant development of laboratory instruments which permit multiple automated tests, use of a battery of chemistry screening tests is common. As noted in Chap. 1, another advantage of these tests is the establishment of base-line normal values for individuals, which can be critical to evaluation if the individual develops an illness.

One of the various automated instruments now in use is the Autoanalyser.[1] The Autoanalyser has been developed into a multiple-

[1]Product of the Technicon Corp., Tarrytown, N.Y.

channel model, with as many as 12 channels for a corresponding number of tests, using a single sample of 2.5 ml serum. This instrument is referred to as the SMA (sequential multiple analysis).[1] (See Fig. 4-1a.) The instrument may be equipped with a print-out mechanism which records the 12 results on a graph form, which includes shaded areas indicating normal ranges, thus making it possible to evaluate results at a glance (see Fig. 4-1b). Individual laboratories may not use this reporting device, however. With the increasing use of computer print-outs which record daily and cumulative results, such a system is unnecessary.

It has become common practice for the physician to request the battery of tests included in these analyses as SMA. The usual tests for screening outpatients are uric acid, inorganic phosphorus, cholesterol, lactic dehydrogenase, total protein, albumin, urea nitrogen, glucose, calcium, bilirubin, alkaline phosphatase, and glutamic oxaloacetic transaminase. Hospital laboratories generally substitute sodium, potassium, chloride, and carbon dioxide for uric acid, phosphorus, cholesterol, and LDH of the screening battery.

CHEMICAL ELEMENTS

Calcium

Abbreviation: Ca
Normal range: 4.8–5.2 meq/liter

Calcium serves in a variety of important biologic processes. It is essential to formation of bony tissue, to muscular activity, and to the blood-coagulation mechanism. Hypocalcemia is seen in rickets, parathyroid tetany, nephrosis, Bright's disease, osteomalacia, and hypoparathyroidism. Hypercalcemia is seen in hyperparathyroidism and osteitis. Calcium is the most common constituent of urinary calculi.

---

[1]SMA is a trademark of the Technicon Corp., Tarrytown, N.Y.

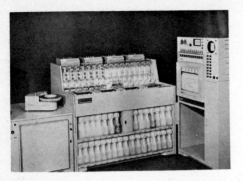

FIG. 4-1a SMA/60, for sequential multiple analyses in chemistry. (*Trademark, Technicon Corp., Tarrytown, N.Y.*)

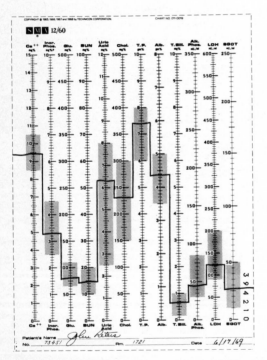

FIG. 4-1b SMA/60-report print-out sheet. Shaded areas in each column indicate normal ranges. Line indicates results obtained on patient's specimen. (*Trademark, Technicon Corp., Tarrytown, N.Y.*)

Copper

Abbreviation: Cu
Normal ranges
  Males: 70–140 μg/dl serum
  Females: 80–155 μg/dl serum

Copper is essential to hemoglobin synthesis, and it participates in respiratory enzymatic activity. About 90 percent of the copper is bound to α_2-globulin, which is ceruloplasmin, the means of transport for copper in the body. Erythrocyte intracellular copper ranges from 90 to 110 μg/dl. In Wilson's disease (hepatolenticular disease), the serum copper level falls to 20 μg/dl and the urinary output may rise to more than 100 μg/24 h. Wilson's disease is marked by tissue deposition of copper, with degeneration of basal ganglia and cirrhosis the most serious results. Radionuclide copper may be used in studies of body retention of copper in suspected cases of Wilson's disease.

Iodine

Determinations of protein-bound iodine and butanol extractable iodine have been used until recently in assessing thyroid function. They are sensitive to contamination by extraneous iodine and are thus subject to error. The methods of choice for thyroid-function assessment are the thyronine and throxin tests using radionuclides of iodine. (See Chap. 12 for these tests.)

Iron

Abbreviation: Fe
Normal range
  Serum iron: 65–170 μg/dl
  Total iron-binding capacity: 250–400 μg/dl

The mechanisms involved in iron uptake for the synthesis of hemoglobin and its return as a result of hemoglobin breakdown are normally well-balanced in relation to dietary intake of iron, maintaining relatively constant levels. In disease, the serum iron level varies according to the characteristics of the disease which affect iron storage and utilization. Decreased serum iron levels are seen when the store of iron is low and the iron intake is insufficient for body requirements. Increased levels occur when available iron exceeds need or when there is impairment of iron utilization.

No special preparation of the patient is required, but glassware, including syringes, used for the test must be chemically clean.

Determination of the capacity of transferrin, the serum protein which binds and transports iron, should be made in conjunction with the serum iron test. Complete saturation of transferrin occurs at about 350 μg/dl serum. Normally, about 30 percent of the transferrin is bound to iron. In iron-deficiency states, the TIBC is increased, whereas excess iron results in a lowered TIBC. This is logical, since in the case of low serum iron levels there is a minimal amount to be bound to transferrin, leaving more available sites for binding. When the serum iron is in excess, a maximal amount of iron is bound to transferrin, markedly reducing its capacity to bind additional iron.

No special preparation of the patient is required, but equipment must be chemically clean, as noted for iron determinations.

Magnesium

   Abbreviation: Mg
   Normal range: 1.6–2.1 meq/liter

Like calcium, magnesium influences muscle activity. It is important in coenzyme activity associated with carbohydrate and protein metabolism. With ordinary diet, the daily requirements for magnesium are readily met. Magnesium deficiency may be seen in malabsorption states and during prolonged intravenous therapy with solutions not containing magnesium.

Inorganic Phosphorus

   Abbreviation: PO_4
   Normal range: 1.7–2.6 meq/liter serum

In addition to its function in osseous-tissue generation, this anion is an important contributor to the metabolism of glucose and to acid-base balance. As phosphorus, it is present in levels roughly half those of calcium. When calcium levels are depressed, the phosphorus level increases and the reverse ratio becomes true, although the relation is not as sensitive. Elevated levels of phosphorus are seen in hypoparathyroidism, uremia, alkalosis, and Bright's disease. Lowered levels are seen in rickets, hyperparathyroidism, osteitis, and osteomalacia.

COMPONENTS OF ACID-BASE BALANCE

Acid-balance is a delicate and intricate interplay of buffer systems, cations and anions, proteins, oxygen, and carbon dioxide. (Fig. 4-2 shows data for body anions and cations in health and disease.) No attempt will be made to simplify these interactions as a whole system. The focus will be on the components contributing to the maintenance of the balance that is essential to life.

Ammonia Nitrogen

Abbreviation: NH_4^+
Normal range: 35–70 μg/dl

Since ammonium, NH_4^+, is a ready source of hydrogen, maintenance of normal levels is critical to acid-base balance. Nitrogen balance is also important, this fraction of ammonium being used to rebuild amino acids. The liver converts ammonia to urea for ready excretion by the kidneys. Hepatic coma may be diagnosed and monitored by ammonia nitrogen determinations. The test is reported in terms of the nitrogen fraction of the ammonia. The test must be performed immediately after drawing the blood.

Carbon Dioxide

Abbreviation: CO_2
Normal range
Content: 24–30 mmol/liter

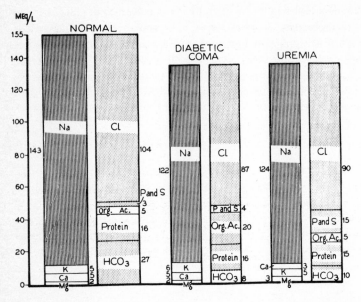

FIG. 4-2 Cation-anion balance in health and disease. (*From W. H. Hoffman, "The Biochemistry of Clinical Medicine," Year Book Medical Publishers, Inc., Chicago, 1954, by permission of the publisher.*)

Combining power: 50–58 vol/dl

Tension (P_{CO_2}): 35–45 mm Hg

A part of the alkali reserve of the body, carbon dioxide reflects the efficiency of the carbonic acid-bicarbonate buffer system. (A buffer is analogous to a chemical sponge. Depending upon the demands made by body conditions, it can "soak up" excess hydrogen ions or release them when needed.) Three measures are possible. Carbon dioxide *content* is the amount of carbonic acid and bicarbonate, reported in millimoles per liter. Carbon dioxide *combining power* refers to the amount of the gas at a given pressure and temperature which will be absorbed; it is reported in terms of volume per deciliter of serum or plasma. Tension is the partial pressure of the gas; it is symbolized as P_{CO_2} and is reported in millimeters of mercury. The test is used to evaluate conditions producing acidosis or alkalosis.

In both these conditions, the underlying cause may be respiratory or metabolic.

In *respiratory acidosis* the pH is lowered, but carbon dioxide is elevated. It is due to (*a*) impairment of air or blood flow to the lungs or (*b*) impairment of carbon dioxide diffusion in the lungs.

In *respiratory alkalosis,* the pH is elevated and carbon dioxide is lowered. It is due to hyperventilation, and, thus, excessive loss of carbon dioxide occurs.

In *metabolic acidosis,* the bicarbonate is decreased, with a corresponding increase in hydrogen-ion concentration, resulting in lowering of both pH and carbon dioxide. Its etiologic pattern may be produced by any of the following three events: (1) ingestion or infusion of acid, which is the most obvious; (2) primary bicarbonate loss resulting from abnormal excretion in the urine (renal-tubular acidosis) or from severe diarrhea; and (3) depletion of the alkali reserve by acid metabolic end products, such as the organic acids that accumulate as a result of deranged carbohydrate metabolism in uncontrolled diabetes mellitus.

In *metabolic alkalosis* both the pH and carbon dioxide are elevated. These changes occur in the extracellular fluid, with intracellular acidosis occurring concomitantly. It results from intake of excessive alkali and from severe vomiting. It is often seen in potassium deficiency.

It is possible to have more than one condition simultaneously. The combination of respiratory and metabolic acidosis is the most common. This condition is serious because the compensating mechanisms of the buffer system are inhibited.

Oxygen

Abbreviation: O_2
Normal range
  Content: 15–23 vol/dl
  Saturation: 95–97%
  Tension (P_{O_2}): 80–90 mm Hg

As would be expected, the in vivo oxygen content of the blood varies with the hemoglobin concentration. Similarly, there is a difference between arterial and venous blood, which reflects the physiologic function of the red blood cells. At standard temperature and pressure, 1.34 ml oxygen combines with 1 g hemoglobin. Tests for oxygen are usually performed on arterial blood.

Four measures of oxygen are possible. Oxygen *content* refers to the in vivo amount present and is reported as volumes per deciliter. Oxygen *capacity* is the maximum amount the blood is capable of holding. *Saturation* is the ratio of content to capacity, reported in percent. *Tension* is the partial pressure of oxygen, reported as P_{O_2} in terms of mm of mercury. Because so many variables can affect values for oxygen (physical activity, age, sex, smoking habits, etc.), it is difficult to establish normal values. As may be expected, measures related to oxygen are useful in evaluation of cardiopulmonary abnormalities. Decreases in saturation and tension are associated with (*a*) impairment of diffusion within the lungs, (*b*) hypoventilation, (*c*) arteriovenous shunt, and (*d*) lack of uniform ventilation in relation to blood flow.

The test should be performed immediately after obtaining the blood specimen.

Blood pH

Normal range: 7.35–7.45 (arterial blood)

This is a measure of the hydrogen-ion concentration in the blood. Differences between arterial and venous blood are noted, but the routine test is done on arterial blood and the values given are for that source. The pH of the blood is maintained within a very narrow range and is the expression of the interaction of the whole battery of elements and buffer systems within the body. Any deviation outside the normal range is serious and can result in death.

Potassium

Abbreviation: K
Normal range: 4.0–5.4 meq/liter

Like sodium, potassium is important in cation-anion balance. Because of its role in electric conductance, it is essential to proper muscular function. It is principally found intracellularly, the overall intracellular concentration being about 23 times that in the extracellular fluid. No one condition specifically results in hyperpotassemia. When present, intoxication of hyperpotassemia is revealed principally in its effect on the heart. High potassium levels disrupt the normal electric conductance of the heart muscle, and, as a consequence, the normal contraction sequence is disturbed. Death may result from potassium intoxication. In hyperpotassemia, characteristic changes are noted in the electrocardiograph. Hypopotassemia is associated with alkalosis, impaired renal function, and marked vomiting. When glucose and/or insulin are administered, a fall of 1.0 meq/liter in the potassium level may occur.

Preparation of the patient may require that the blood sample be obtained when the patient is in the fasting state, although this is not absolutely necessary. The blood is drawn carefully so as to avoid hemolysis.

Sodium

Abbreviation: Na
Normal range: 136–142 meq/liter blood
Source of blood: venipuncture

Sodium is extremely important in water balance because of its large contribution to the essential cation-anion balance and its effect on osmotic pressures. It is also essential to the acid-base balance. Low sodium levels (hyponatremia) are seen in diabetic coma, dehydration, uremia, severe diarrhea, Addison's disease, and pyloric obstruction. High sodium levels (hypernatremia) are uncommon but, when seen, are associated with coma. Hypernatremia may result from impaired renal function, increased adrencortical activity, and brain injury involving the hypothalamus and/or posterior pituitary.

ENZYMES

The suffix *-ase* indicates an enzyme. Enzymes are catalytic agents that promote biochemical processes. Their activity is influenced by the hydrogen-ion concentration (each has an optimal, specific pH range) and by temperature. Since they are protein in nature, their separation by electrophoresis is possible.

Subsequent to the discovery of the primary biologic enzymes, further investigation revealed that, in many instances, enzymes fall into groups of isoenzymes, i.e., enzymes with the same functional effect but different in structural and physical characteristics. Assays of organs (and, in some cases, structures within organs) have revealed differences in isoenzyme content; these differences are sufficiently characteristic to aid in identification of the source of pathologic conditions. Patterns of enzymes also contribute to identification of sites of disease. Testing for selected enzyme levels may be used to monitor tissue rejection in organ transplants.

When a tissue undergoes damage (trauma, infection, infarction, etc.), the tissue loses significant amounts of cytoplasmic isoenzymes into the circulating blood, so that the peripheral blood pattern represents a composite of the enzymes normally present in the blood combined and those derived from damaged tissue. Tumor-tissue assays are especially valuable in identifying the primary source of metastatic malignancy. For this purpose, the sample of tissue must be preserved by freezing, *without* being exposed to the usual fixative fluids such as Formalin.

The enzyme tests discussed below are those which are the most commonly used in daily practice. Many more have been developed, but they may not be used, either because they offer little additional information that is useful clinically or because they are still in the investigative stages, awaiting evaluation of their clinical usefulness and practicality.

Acid Phosphatase

Abbreviation: ac phos
Normal range: 1.0–4.0 King-Armstrong units

This enzyme is optimally active at pH 5.0 to 6.0; hence the name *acid* phosphatase. It is present in many types of cells in the body, especially in the prostate gland. Its function in this area is thought to be related to the activity of spermatozoa in the female genital tract. Normally the prostatic secretions remove the acid phosphatase from the body. But when metastatic carcinoma of the prostate is present, cells that produce the enzyme become walled off from the ducts that drain the secretion to the exterior, and the level of serum acid phosphatase rises accordingly. The test is useful, therefore, in the diagnosis of prostatic carcinoma.

Alkaline Phosphatase

Abbreviation: alk phos
Normal range: 2.0–5.0 Bodansky units

Alkaline phosphatase is an enzyme which hydrolyses phosphate esters in an alkaline medium (the optimal pH being 8.5 to 9.5), releasing inorganic phosphorus. The unit refers to the enzyme activity required to raise the inorganic phosphorus level by one milligram under specified conditions of pH, time, and temperature. Tissues rich in the various isoenzymes of the alkaline-phosphatase group are:

Type	Tissue
1	Liver
2	Bone
3	Intestine
4	Kidney
5	Placenta

Alkaline phosphatase levels are high in the proximal convoluted tubules of the kidney, growing bone, bile canaliculi, and the lactating breast. The test is useful in evaluation of the status of pregnancy because type 5 reflects the function of the placenta. The principal use of the test is in evaluation of liver and bone disease.

Aldolase

Abbreviation: ald
Normal range

TABLE 4-1   CONDITIONS ASSOCIATED WITH ELEVATIONS
OF ALKALINE PHOSPHATASE

Isoenzyme type	Condition
Liver	Obstructive jaundice, metastatic tumors to liver, hepatitis
Bone	Osteogenic sarcoma, Paget's disease, metastatic carcinoma to the bone (breast, prostate, etc.)
Intestinal	Perforation, ulcerative disease, pregnancy
Kidney	Renal infarct, tissue rejection
Placenta	Pregnancy

Adults: 3–8 Sibley-Lehninger units/dl
Children: about three times that of adults

This enzyme is most useful in monitoring diseases affecting skeletal muscle, such as muscular dystrophy, dermatomyositis, and trichinosis. Other conditions in which elevated levels are noted include myocardial infarction, hepatic necrosis, carcinomatosis, and granulocytic leukemia. Aldolase is a glycolytic enzyme which catalyzes the cleavage of fructose 1, 6-diphosphate into glyceraldehyde phosphate and dihydroxyacetone phosphate.

Amylase

Abbreviation: none used
Normal range: 60–150 Somogyi units

Amylase is secreted by the pancreas. Its substrate (compound upon which it acts) is starch. Elevation of amylase levels is seen in acute pancreatitis. Serial determinations are valuable in evaluating the progress of the disease. The results are reported in units, which express the amount of starch hydrolyzed under prescribed conditions of temperature, pH, and time. No special preparation of the patient is required. In fact, it is important to obtain the blood sample during an acute attack.

Cholinesterase

Abbreviation: ChE
Normal range: 0.5–1.0 pH unit

Hydrolysis of acetylcholine to choline and acetic acid is catalyzed by this enzyme. Two forms have been identified: "true" cholinesterase and pseudocholinesterase. The former is found in nerve tissue and red blood cells; the latter in the serum. The primary use of the test is in evaluating overexposure to insecticides containing organic phosphorous compounds. Patients with hereditary atypical cholinesterase are particularly sensitive to muscle relaxants such as succinyl choline, manifested by prolonged apnea following use of the drug.

Creatine Phosphokinase

Abbreviation: CPK
Normal range: 0–200 sigma units

Creatine phosphokinase catalyzes the phosphorylation of creatine by adenosine triphosphate. There are four isoenzymes in this group. The highest concentration of CPK is found in skeletal muscles. The principal uses of the test are in diagnosis of Duchenne-Aran muscular dystrophy and differential diagnosis of myocardial infarction (see Table 4-2). Special note should be taken of the fact that falsely elevated levels occur following intramuscular injections and surgery. In the latter case, 24 to 48 h are required to clear the circulation of CPK released as a result of the trauma of surgery.

Lactic Acid Dehydrogenase

Abbreviation: LDH
Normal range: 165–300 units

There are five isoenzymes of LDH, all of which accomplish the catalytic action necessary to remove hydrogen ions from lactic acid

TABLE 4-2   SUMMARY OF ISOENZYME PATTERNS
(Numbers refer to isoenzymes within a group)

Condition	Alkaline phosphatase	LDH	CPK
Infectious hepatitis	1	5	
Infectious mononucleosis	1	5	
Obstructive jaundice	1	5	
Acute yellow atrophy	1	4, 5	
Myocardial infarct		1, 2*	2, 3**
Pulmonary infarct		3, 4	
Hemolysis		1, 2	
Sickle cell anemia		3, 4, 5	
Megaloblastic anemia		1	
Meningitis (supporative)		3, 4, 5	
Meningitis (nonsupporative)		2, 3, 4	
Brain tumor		1, 2, 3	1
Cerebrovascular accident			1
Acute pancreatitis		3, 4, 5	
Acute glomerulonephritis	4	4, 5	
Dermatomyositis		5	
Pregnancy	5	4, 5	
Muscular dystrophy		3, 4, 5	2, 3
Malignancy	Increases associated with primary site and metastatic involvement of other organs.		

*Slow rise and fall.
**Rapid rise and fall.

to produce pyruvic acid. Each LDH isoenzyme is a tetramer made up of various combinations of subunits referred to as H (heart) and M (voluntary muscle). The two subunits combine in various proportions to form the five LDH isoenzymes, as shown in Table 4-3.

The principal uses of LDH determinations are in differential diagnosis of myocardial infarction, pulmonary infarction and liver disease. There are detailed descriptions of patterns of isoenzymes associated with each. (See Table 4-2 for highlights of these details.) An example of quality control in enzyme determinations is shown in the association of markedly elevated LDH-5 levels when there is diffuse skin disease (dermatomyositis). Information about this

TABLE 4-3   TETRAMERS OF LDH ISOENZYMES

Isoenzyme	Tetramer
LDH-1	H H H H (pure heart fraction)
LDH-2	H H H M
LDH-3	H H M M
LDH-4	H M M M
LDH-5	M M M M (pure muscle fraction)

skin condition should be included on the requisition so that appropriate interpretation of results is possible.

In myocardial infarction, the LDH-1, -2 levels peak and subside relatively slowly, in contrast to CPK, which peaks and subsides rapidly. Serial determinations are essential to adequate monitoring of the disease process. It should also be noted that sequential events secondary to the primary disease have an effect. For example, in myocardial infarction with shock, there is marked elevation of LDH-4, -5 due to extensive necrosis of the central liver lobules secondary to severe anoxia (see also Table 4-4).

In pulmonary infarct, LDH-3 is elevated, but it should be noted that since hemorrhage is common, some masking of results is possible

TABLE 4-4   DISTRIBUTION OF LDH ISOENZYMES
IN ORGANS

Organ	Structure	LDH isoenzyme(s)
Liver	Cells adjacent to central veins	4
	All areas	5
Kidney	Cortex, medulla	1, 2
	Inferior medullary pyramid, papillae	4
Heart	Intraventricular septum	1
	Anterior ventricular wall	1, 2
	Right heart	5
	Apex	1, 2
Lung	All areas	3

if only the total LDH is measured. There may be mild elevation of LDH-5 because of associated passive congestion of the liver.

In infectious hepatitis, marked elevation of LDH-5 and moderate elevation of LDH-4 occur. These elevations occur before clinical jaundice is detected. Return to normal levels marks progress in convalescence, even though jaundice persists. Infectious mononucleosis with liver involvement may give rise to LDH-5, and if the spleen is also involved, LDH-2, -3, and -4 will also rise. Drug and toxic effects on the liver are monitored by LDH-5. For example, chlorpromazine can produce high levels of LDH-5, even though the patient appears well. Carbon tetrachloride poisoning produces very high levels of LDH-5.

LDH-4, -5 are found in secretions of the amnion, and determinations of these levels during pregnancy can be a valuable means of assessing placental viability.

Lipase

Abbreviation: none used
Normal range
Cherry and Crandall method: 1.0–1.5 units
Maclay method: less than 0.3 units

This enzyme is secreted by the pancreas and functions in fat digestion. The lipase level is elevated in acute pancreatitis and returns to normal levels more slowly than does the amylase level. The results of the test are expressed as the amount of sodium hydroxide required to neutralize the fatty acids produced by the action of the lipase contained in 1 ml serum on the olive-oil substrate used. Cherry and Crandall method requires 24-h incubation, and the Maclay modification requires incubation for 1 h.

Transaminases

Normal range
Serum glutamic-oxaloacetic transaminase (SGOT): 10–40 units
Serum glutamic-pyruvic transaminase (SGPT): 5–35 units

The first enzyme catalyzes the transfer of the amino radical (NH_2) from glutamic acid to oxaloacetic acid to form aspartic acid (SGOT); the second enzyme, from glutamic acid to pyruvic acid to form alanine (SGPT). These enzymes are present in many tissues. The principal uses of these tests are in the differential diagnosis of hepatic and cardiac disease. Serial determinations are important in order to establish a clear picture. Table 4-5 describes the relative elevations associated with liver diseases and myocardial infarction.

LIPIDS

Cholesterol

Abbreviation: chol
Normal range: 150–250 mg/dl

Cholesterol is an alcohol derived from the catabolism of fats. It is also a constituent of many foods. Evaluation of a tendency toward atherosclerosis is aided by information from the cholesterol levels, in combination with other findings. It has been implicated as one of the factors predisposing to myocardial infarction.

Cholesterol esters are the basic cholesterol molecule modified at one carbon to combine with a radical of long-chain fatty acids.

TABLE 4-5   TRANSAMINASE ELEVATIONS ASSOCIATED WITH
LIVER AND HEART DISEASE

Disease	SGOT	SGPT
Infectious hepatitis	Marked	Very marked
Obstructive jaundice	Marked	Moderate
Cholangiolitic hepatitis	Moderate	Marked
Laennec's cirrhosis	Moderate	Slight
Postnectotic cirrhosis	Marked	Moderate
Toxic hepatitis	Marked	Very marked
Infectious mononucleosis	Marked	Very marked
Myocardial infarct	Marked*	Slight

*The levels show a rapid rise and fall.

Total cholesterol is made up of free (i.e., unesterified) and esterified molecules. Since the liver has a prominent role in the metabolism of cholesterol, including its esterification, these compounds are tested for as part of liver function tests. Blood for cholesterol determinations must be obtained in the fasting state.

Triglycerides

Abbreviation: none used
Normal range: 10–190 mg/dl

Triglycerides are tri–esters of glycerol and fatty acids synthesized by the liver utilizing dietary or endogenous carbohydrates; they are also the product of fat digestion. Triglycerides are transported in the bloodstream as pre-β-lipoproteins, substances which are discussed in the next section. Those that have been newly absorbed from the digestive tract are called *chlyomicrons*. Chylomicrons are minute (less than 1 μm in diameter) fat droplets which are covered by a film of protein. Chylomicrons account for the degree of turbidity in serum or plasma following a meal rich in fats, but their appearance in a fasting specimen is abnormal. The turbidity may range from milky to creamy in appearance. When the serum or plasma is turbid, this information should be noted on reports to signal the need for follow-up studies using the lipid panel tests (cholesterol, triglycerides, and lipoprotein electrophoresis). Triglycerides are now considered of greater importance than cholesterol in the etiology of arterial disease.

LIPOPROTEINS

Lipoproteins include the lipid fractions of serum (phospholipids, cholesterol, and triglycerides), all of which are transported in the blood combined with serum proteins. In combination with chemical analysis for cholesterol and triglycerides, lipoprotein electrophoresis is extremely valuable in identification of individuals who are likely to develop atherosclerosis and/or coronary disease. This serves the purposes of preventive medicine very well. Diagnostic use is also made in evaluation of hyperlipoproteinemia which is secondary to other diseases such as diabetes and pancreatitis. The types of hyperlipoproteinemia described below are primarily a reflection of genetic differences, although they may also be acquired as a consequence of some other primary disease.

Precise quantitation of lipoproteins is not necessary, for more useful information is obtained from the electrophoretic patterns which separate α-, β-, and pre-β-lipoproteins. (See Fig. 4-3.)

Type I. Familial hyperproteinemia
Cholesterol slightly elevated; triglycerides markedly elevated; glucose tolerance normal; plasma creamy in appearance; fat inducible.

Type II. Familial hyperprebetalipoproteinemia
Cholesterol moderately elevated; triglycerides upper limits of normal; glucose tolerance normal; plasma clear.

Type III. Hyperlipoproteinemia
Cholesterol markedly elevated; triglycerides moderately elevated; glucose tolerance abnormal; plasma clear to milky; carbohydrate inducible. Xanthochromatosis, ischemic heart disease, and mild diabetes are frequently associated.

Type IV. Familial hyperbetalipoproteinemia
Cholesterol slightly elevated; triglycerides moderately elevated;

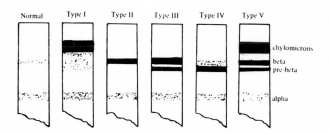

FIG. 4-3 Summary of lipoprotein patterns in familial hyperlipoproteinemia. *(Courtesy of S. T. Nerenberg, M.D., Ph.D., Director, University of Illinois Hospital Laboratories.)*

glucose tolerance abnormal; plasma clear to milky; carbo-hydrate inducible. This is the most common type of hyper-lipoproteinemia. It often develops secondary to diabetes or pancreatitis. It may also be found in patients who are taking contraceptive drugs or are pregnant. Hyperuricemia may be associated with this type.

Type V. Familial hyperchylomicronemia with hyperprebeta-lipoproteinemia
  Cholesterol slightly elevated; triglycerides moderately elevated, with increase in chylomicron concentration; glucose tolerance abnormal; plasma creamy; fat or carbohydrate inducible.

Preparation of the patient for lipid panel studies requires the fasting state, normal diet for at least 2 weeks, no alcoholic beverages for 24 to 48 h, and no recent radiologic examinations using contrast media. The screening panel includes determinations of cholesterol, triglycerides, and a lipoprotein pherogram. Because elevated uric acid and diabetes mellitus (occult or frank) are commonly associated with types III, IV, and V, uric acid and a 2-h postprandial glucose should be determined if hyperlipemia is revealed.

Hypolipoproteinemia occurs in familial diseases in which there is a lack of β-lipoprotein or α-lipoprotein. In the latter (Tangier disease), the heterozygous person has lower than normal α-lipo-protein, and in the homozygous person it is virtually absent.

Diseases with which hyperlipoproteinemia may be associated as a secondary disease include the following:

Diabetes	Nephrotic syndrome
Pancreatitis	Abnormal plasma globulins
Alcoholism	Obstructive liver disease
Glycogen storage disease	Obesity
Hypothyroidism	Myocardial infarct

As noted above, contraceptive drugs and pregnancy also may pro-duce hyperlipoproteinemia of type IV. In the latter, the hyperlipo-proteinemia subsides within 2 to 3 months following delivery.

NONPROTEIN NITROGEN COMPOUNDS

Nonprotein nitrogenous compounds are small-molecule crystalloids of the body fluids, particularly of blood and urine; they include amino acids (the building blocks of proteins) as well as substances such as urea. Proteins and nucleic acids are macromolecules and, though they contain nitrogen in their structures, are not included in this group of compounds. As a whole, nonprotein nitrogenous compounds are present in the blood at levels of 10 to 40 mg/dl. The NPN test, which indicaets the total amount of nonprotein nitrogenous compounds, was used in the past, but it has fallen into disuse because the constituent compounds assessed separately are better measures of clinical significance.

Creatine, Creatinine

Abbreviation: creat
Normal range: 0.5–1.2 mg/dl blood

Creatine, synthesized from glycine and parts of arginine and methionine, is present in high concentrations in muscle as phosphocreatine, a rich source of high-energy-phosphate storage. Creatinine is an anhydride of creatine and is the primary excretory product of creatine. Creatinine is readily excreted by the kidneys; whereas creatine is reabsorbed to a high degree. Elevation of the creatinine level (in the absence of muscular activity, since creatine is proportional to muscle mass) indicates kidney shutdown.

Urea Nitrogen

Abbreviation: BUN (blood urea nitrogen)
Normal range: 8–28 mg/dl blood

One of the major nonprotein nitrogenous substances, urea is also a major excretory product of the kidney. The test determines the nitrogen fraction of the compound, as the name indicates. Results are reported in terms of the nitrogen fraction, although it is a simple matter to calculate for the entire compound by multiplying the nitrogen fraction by a factor of 2.14. Diseases of the kidney and diseases that affect kidney function produce elevated levels of urea.

Uric Acid

Abbreviation: none used
Normal range: 3.0–5.0 mg/dl blood

Uric acid is an end product of the metabolism of a class of compounds known as purine bodies. When an abundance of uric acid crystals in the tophi of gout was observed, attention was drawn to using the uric acid test as a diagnostic aid in this disease, although it is not specific. It is also used to gauge the prognosis in eclampsia, since it reflects the extent of liver damage in true toxemia of pregnancy.

PIGMENTS

Bilirubin

Alternate test name: van den Bergh
Normal range
   Total: 0.1–1.2 mg/dl serum
   Direct: 0.05–1.4 mg/dl serum
   Indirect: 0.4–0.8 mg/dl serum

Bilirubin is the product of hemoglobin catabolism. Direct bilirubin refers to that which is conjugated with glucuronide and soluble in water; indirect, to that which is not conjugated (free) and not soluble in water. These characteristics facilitate separation of the two fractions.

Since bilirubin undergoes conjugation in the liver, this test is an important measure of liver function. It is also of critical importance in evaluating hemolytic anemias. For example, in neonatal hemolytic anemia or congenital kernicterus, the decision to perform an exchange transfusion depends on the bilirubin level. Normal range for total bilirubin in the neonatal period is 1 to 12 mg/dl. Kernicterus, which occurs when bilirubin levels are high and the blood-brain barrier (as in infants) is not fully developed, results in brain damage which may lead to mental retardation.

Myoglobin

Myoglobin is a protein component of fluids in skeletal muscle. After rapid destruction of skeletal muscle, as in trauma or excessive exercise, myoglobin is excreted in the urine, giving it a pink to red-brown color. It may be differentiated from hemoglobin and other substances imparting these colors to the urine by chemical tests or spectroscopy.

PLASMA AND SERUM PROTEINS

The routine tests for serum proteins include those for total protein, albumin, and total globulin fractions. In addition to chemical determinations of protein levels, electrophoresis is used to study proteins. This process separates the various protein fractions by means of an electric current flowing through the serum-buffer solution on a cellulose acetate supporting medium. The protein fractions migrate under these conditions of pH and electric current in characteristic direction and speed. The direction and rate of migration are functions of the molecular size and charge of the proteins. Direction is toward either the cathode or the anode electric poles. Electrophoretic studies are invaluable in the study of many diseases in which distribution and/or amounts of protein constituents are altered. It is also used to separate the various major human hemoglobins, such as hemoglobins A, C, and S.

After separation by electrophoresis, the specimen is stained, and the relative amounts of the various serum proteins are determined with the use of a densitometer. Normal ranges are given below.

Protein	Range, g/dl serum
Total	6.5–8.0
Albumin	4.0–5.5
α_1-Globulin	0.1–0.4
α_2-Globulin	0.4–1.2
β-Globulin	0.5–1.1
γ-Globulin	0.5–1.6

Figure 4-4 shows the normal distribution of serum proteins when separated by electrophoresis and stained. Table 4-6 shows some typical serum protein patterns of distribution in normal and disease states.

Further separation of the globulins may be done using immuno-logic precipitin reactions with electrophoresis and by radioimmune

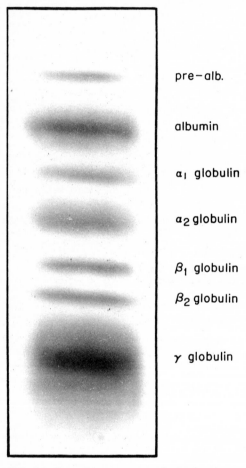

FIG. 4-4 Normal human serum electrophoretogram.

TABLE 4-6   TYPICAL SERUM PROTEIN PATTERNS
IN NORMAL AND DISEASE STATES

Conditions	Total protein	Albumin	α-Globulin	β-Globulin	γ-Globulin
Normal	100% (6.5–8.0 g/dl)	53%	14%	12%	20%
Acute and chronic nephritis	Usually normal	Slight decrease	Slight decrease	Normal	Slight to moderate increase
Cirrhosis	Decrease	Decrease	Frequent decrease	Slight increase	Increase
Collagen vascular diseases	Usually normal	Decrease	Increase	Normal to slight increase or decrease	Increase
Hepatitis	Usually normal	Decrease	Slight decrease	Slight decrease	Increase
Infections and inflammations (liver normal)	Usually normal	Usually normal	Increase	Bacterial infection: marked increase Viral infection: slight increase	Increase
Malignant diseases & leukemia	Normal	Decrease	Slight increase	Slight increase	Slight increase
Myeloma	Usually increased	Usually increased	Myeloma protein may be present in any of the globulin fractions and may be as much as 80% of the total protein		
Nephrosis	Decreased	Great decrease	Great decrease	Normal to slight decrease	Slight to moderate decrease
Obstructive jaundice (early)	Normal	Normal	Normal	Normal	Normal

assay. In precipitin reactions, antigen (the unknown globulin fraction) and antibody (against known globulin fraction) are placed in an agar medium. If the unknown specimen contains the protein corresponding to the known antibody, a zone pf precipitation of antigen-antibody complex forms. In radioimmune assay, specific antibodies which are tagged with an appropriate radionuclide are reacted with the unknown sample, and identification-quantification are based on counts of radioactive particles discharged by the radionuclide.

Albumin

The primary plasma/serum protein constituent is albumin, with molecular weight of 69,000, which is synthesized by the liver. It contributes heavily to the osmotic pressure of blood and acts as a carrier medium for substances which are minimally soluble in water, such as bilirubin, fatty acids, hormones, and drugs. These substances are considered "soluble" in serum or plasma, but this is more apparent than real, since they form loosely bound complexes with albumin. When such substances are analyzed by fractions termed "bound" and "free," reference is to that which is attached or not attached to the protein molecule. Being the smallest of protein molecules, albumin is the most easily lost via damaged renal structures.

Fibrinogen

Fibrinogen, normally present in amounts of 200 to 400 mg/dl *plasma,* is the precursor to fibrin, which forms the blood clot. Obviously, plasma must be used for determination of levels of this important protein. Low levels may be associated with hepatic dysfunction, since the liver is the site of synthesis of fibrinogen. The principal coagulopathy in which low levels of fibrinogen are found is disseminated intravascular coagulation (see Chap. 3).

Globulins

Unlike the homologous character of albumin, the globulin fraction is a family of different proteins. The globulins are similar in electrophoretic mobilities but different chemical structures. Some of the globules serve as transport media; others are antibodies.

α_1-*Globulin* is important in lipid and hormone transport. Hormone globulins found in this fraction are transcortin (cortisol-binding) and thyroid-binding globulin (TBG). Glycoproteins are also in this fraction.

α_2-*Globulins* include many glycoproteins. Ceruloplasmin (the copper-globulin complex) and haptoglobulin (hemoglobin-globulin complex) also migrate in this fraction. Haptoglobulin binds hemoglobin released from erythrocytes and is taken up by reticuloendothelial cells, where degradation of hemoglobin occurs. The enzymes lactic acid dehydrogenase and alkaline phosphatase migrate to the α_2-globulin electrophoretic zone.

β-Globulins include β-liproproteins; hemopexin (binds heme but not hemoglobin); plasminogen (precursor to plasmin, which lyses fibrin); transferrin (iron-globulin complex); and complement.

The *γ-globulin* fraction is the family of antibodies, as indicated by the notation Ig (immunoglobulin). Normal ranges for the immunoglobulins are given below:

Immunoglobulin	Range, mg/dl serum
IgG	800–1,600
IgA	50–250
IgM	40–120
IgD	0.5–3.0
IgE	0.01–0.04

γ-Globulins are produced by plasmacytes and lymphocytes. B-cell lymphocytes (bursa-dependent) produce humoral antibodies; T-cell lymphocytes (thymus-dependent) produce antibodies in cell-mediated immunity. Humoral antibodies are those which are active against bacteria, viruses, etc. and circulate in body fluids. Cell-mediated immunity is that which is primarily fixed to given cells; it is found in such conditions as atopy, transplant rejection, and intracellular microorganism infections. As expected, the patient with agammaglobulinemia or hypogammaglobulinemia is highly susceptible to infections.

An additional distinction which may be made among the γ-globulins is that between monoclonal and polyclonal sources. In monoclonal, the globulin is that produced by a line of lymphocytes or plasmacytes derived from a single parent cell, resulting in only one type of globulin. Monoclonal γ-globulins are seen in myeloma and macroglobulinemia. In these diseases, the plasma cell or immuno-logically competent lymphocyte proliferates and produces the characteristic γ-globulin without an external stimulus. Polyclonal γ-globulins are the product of many clones of cells, with a diffuse increase in antibody proteins. Examples of conditions giving rise to polyclonal γ-globulins are chronic infections, granulomatous diseases, collagen disease, and autoimmune disease.

Cryoglobulins have been so designated because they precipitate out of the serum when the temperature is reduced to about $4°C$, return into the colloidal state on warming. They are found in the IgG group primarily; occasionally, in the IgM group. Cryoglobulins are not normally present. They are associated with a wide variety of diseases.

Macroglobulins are characteristically found in multiple myeloma and Waldenstrom's syndrome. The Bence Jones protein of myeloma is the most common. γ-Globulin molecular weights range from 160,000 to 200,000. Macroglobulins may have molecular weights as high as 1 million. This gammopathy may also be associated with lymphoma and lymphatic leukemia.

SUGARS

Galactose

Galactosemia is an inherited disease in which there is a deficiency of galactose 1-phosphate uridyl transferase. Liver damage and mental retardation, as well as cataracts, are the result of this disease. These may be prevented by careful control of diet early in life. Diagnosis is based on chromatographic identification of the sugar after finding a positive copper-reduction (e.g., Clinitest[1])

[1] Clinitest and Dextrostix are the products of Ames Company, Elkhart, Ind.

test of urine and a negative glucose oxidase test of urine.

Glucose

Abbreviation: gluc
Alternate name: blood sugar
Normal range: 65–120 mg/dl in the fasting state
                  (Somogyi-Nelson method)

Preparation of the patient for a routine blood glucose determination requires that he be fasting. Diabetic patients should not receive their dose of insulin until after the blood specimen is obtained. There may be times when the physician needs to know the patient's response to food intake and will order a blood glucose determination to be done at a specified time after a meal. This is usually 2 h postprandially. In requesting this test, it should be noted whether it is to be drawn while the patient is fasting or at a specific time of day.

A simple semiquantitative test for glucose may be performed using the Dextrostix[1] test. This test requires but a drop of blood, which may be obtained from a finger puncture. It distinguishes low, medium (normal range), and high levels. Care must be taken to follow the directions explicitly.

Glucose Tolerance

Time required
  Standard test: 4–5 h
  Exton-Rose test: 1½ h

Glucose-tolerance tests are done to determine the patient's response to a standard amount of glucose. These tests are of value in ruling out diabetes mellitus and in diagnosing hyperinsulinism.

STANDARD AND EXTON-ROSE TESTS

Two different forms of glucose-tolerance tests are available. The standard test (in which 100 g glucose is given in a single dose

[1] Clinitest and Dextrostix are the products of Ames Company, Elkhart, Ind.

and specimens are collected hourly for 4 to 5 h) is most generally used. The Exton-Rose test (a 1 h two-dose test) is limited to the diagnosis of diabetes mellitus, since it is completed before a reaction of hyperinsulinism could take place.

Preparation of the Patient

1. Blood and urine specimens are obtained with the patient in the fasting state ½ h after ingestion of glucose and each hour thereafter for the required time. The urine specimens need not be large in amount, since only a partial analysis of each is made.
2. No food is to be eaten during the test period.
3. Water is allowed ad lib. The patient is encouraged to drink water in order that urine specimens may be obtained when indicated. No coffee, tea, etc. is allowed during the test period.
4. No smoking is allowed during the test period, since smoking produces physiologic stimulation that may alter the results.
5. The patient should not leave his room during the test period. This is to make sure that he is available at the proper times and to minimize exercise, which could affect the glucose level.

The glucose is dissolved in water and flavored with lemon juice to make it more palatable. However, some persons find it difficult to take a sweet preparation without previous food. The patient should be encouraged to drink the glucose solution as quickly as possible. The entire amount must be taken, since the test is based on the ingestion of a specific amount of glucose. Commercial preparations containing the proper amount of glucose for the standard test are now available. These preparations are Glucola[1] and Gel-a-dex.[2] Glucola is a carbonated drink, and Gel-a-dex is cherry-flavored gelatin. When these products are used, the patient is given a palatable form of the 100-g glucose load, overcoming both psychologic and physiologic side effects.

[1] Glucola is the product of the Ames Company, Elkhart, Ind.
[2] Gel-a-dex is the product of Unitech, Sun Valley, Calif.

Possible Reactions

One might expect the patient to have some psychologic reaction to as many as six venipunctures performed in 4 h. This varies with the patient's attitude. If he faints readily while having venipunctures done, an outpatient should be put to bed if possible.

Sometimes, between the second and third hours, the patient may develop weakness, giddiness, and sweating. This is probably caused by a fall in the blood glucose level to below the fasting level, secondary to the increased secretion of insulin, which is the normal response to elevated glucose levels. The reaction is transitory unless hyperinsulinism is involved. All such reactions should be recorded.

Procedure for Standard Test

1. The patient is fed a high-carbohydrate diet for 3 days preceding test.
2. Start the test with the patient in the fasting state.
3. Draw blood with the patient in the fasting state and ½, 1, 2, 3, 4 (and more, if indicated) h after the ingestion of 100 g glucose in water. Mark all specimens with the time drawn.
4. After obtaining the fasting specimen, give the patient the glucose solution to drink. He must drink the entire amount. Note time he finishes drinking the solution and collect specimens at intervals indicated in Table 4-7. Collect urine specimens on the same schedule.
5. Allow water ad lib but no food or smoking during the test period.

Procedure for Exton-Rose Test

1. The patient is fed a high-carbohydrate diet for 3 days preceding test.
2. Start the test with the patient in the fasting state.
3. Obtain blood and urine samples during the fasting state.
4. Give the patient 50 g glucose in solution to drink. He must drink the entire amount. Note the time he finishes drinking the solution.

TABLE 4-7   TYPICAL VALUES IN GLUCOSE-TOLERANCE TESTS
(All results given in mg/dl blood)

Condition	Fasting	30 min	60 min	120 min	180 min
Standard test					
Normal	80	150	135	100	80
Diabetic	160	250	300	380	290
Mild diabetic	130	200	280	225	180
Hyperinsulinism	80	95	50	60	70

Condition	Specimen	Fasting	½ h	1 h
Exton-Rose test				
Normal	Blood	80	150	160
	Urine	Neg	Neg	Neg
Diabetic	Blood	130	225	250
	Urine	Neg	Variable	Pos

5. Obtain blood and urine samples ½ h after the first dose of glucose is taken.
6. Give the patient a second dose of 50 g glucose in solution to drink immediately after the ½-h samples of blood and urine have been collected. Note the time.
7. Collect blood and urine samples ½ h after the second dose of glucose solution.
8. Allow water ad lib but no food or smoking during the test period.

POSTPRANDIAL GLUCOSE DETERMINATIONS

An increasingly common procedure being used as a simple screening test is the 2-h postprandial blood glucose determination, which may indicate an abnormally high level in persons with diabetic tendency. Its value as a screening test would be markedly enhanced if, as studies have shown, the patient is given a meal with known carbohydrate quantities rather than a random diet. A result greater than 120 mg/dl is considered indicative and should be followed with further tests to confirm a diagnosis of diabetes mellitus.

TOXICOLOGY AND DRUG EVALUATIONS

Many toxicologic tests are complicated and require techniques that are frequently not feasible for the usual clinical laboratory. However, some screening tests are available, and these are increasingly being added to the repertoire of the clinical laboratory. Since toxicology is frequently related to legal proceedings, it is important to note the exact time of collection of specimens and to be absolutely certain in the identification of specimens. Gonzales points out five important factors that help the toxicologist to organize his investigation of materials for analysis:

1. Case history
2. Clinical symptoms
3. Testimony of witnesses
4. Extraneous evidence found at the scene
5. Pathologic findings

In forensic medicine, it is just as important to rule out guilt as it is to establish grounds for prosecution. In addition, insurance companies often need certain information.

Evaluation of drug levels is important in monitoring treatment, as well as in toxicologic situations. This section, therefore, combines these two considerations.

Alcohols

ETHANOL

In most instances, determination of blood alcohol level is associated with investigation of traffic accidents in which drunkeness is suspected to be a contributing factor. As a legal proceeding, the note about marking the time when the specimen was drawn is especially critical in these cases. In preparing the site for venipuncture, some antiseptic other than ethanol must be used, since there could be damagingly erroneous results obtained because of extraneous alcohol contaminating the specimen. While there are individual differences in tolerance for alcohol, studies have shown that there is a corresponding range of concentrations associated with observable symptoms, as given below.

TABLE 4-8   BLOOD ALCOHOL LEVELS

Range	mg/dl	Symptoms
0.01–0.05	10–50	None apparent
0.05–0.1	50–100	Stereoscopic vision and adaptation to dark may be affected
0.1–0.15	100–159	Euphoria; reaction time and inhibitions affected
0.15–2.0	150–200	Reaction time markedly affected; slight to moderate effect on equilibrium and coordination
0.2–0.25	200–250	Equilibrium and coordination disturbed; cloudy consciousness
0.35–0.4	350–400	Coma; possibly death

METHANOL

Known as methyl alcohol, or more commonly, as wood alcohol, this alcohol may be used in antifreeze, for example. Its poisonous effect, in addition to the possibility of death, is blindness, which can occur after a single dose or after a series of small doses. Severe poisoning culminates in convulsions and respiratory failure. The danger level is reached at about 80 mg/dl blood.

Amphetamines

Included in this category of drugs are amphetamine, dextro-amphetamine, and methamphetamine, which stimulate the central nervous system. In a therapeutic sense, they have limited use, but they are important because of abuse. They interact with natural inhibitors sufficiently to release large amounts of norepinephrine at the nerve endings, which may result in a hypertensive crisis. Correlations between "safe" levels and toxic levels with respect to symptoms have not been completed. Thin-layer chromatography is required to detect amphetamines.

Barbiturates

Therapeutic level (antiepileptic control): 10–40 μg/ml blood
Toxic levels
Short-acting: 3 mg/dl blood
Long-acting: 9 mg/dl blood

In cases of suspected overdose, blood, urine, or gastric contents may be examined for screening purposes. At least 5 ml of specimen is required. For quantitative analysis, blood is the best specimen.

Bromides

Toxic levels: 100–200 mg/dl blood

Being in the same chemical class (halides) as chlorides, but more active, bromides displace chlorides in the body fluids and cells. This results in central nervous system depression at sufficiently elevated concentrations, with variation among individual responses. Alcoholics are more sensitive to this drug. In otherwise unexplainable neurologic symptoms, a test for bromide can be useful, since it is a common component of proprietary drugs.

Carbon Monoxide

Toxic level: 25% saturation of hemoglobin

Carbon monoxide combines with heme, forming a complex that is 200 times stronger than that between heme and oxygen. Its toxic effect is anoxemia. In the presence of anemia, less than 25 percent saturation is required to produce toxic effects.

Digitoxin, Digoxin

Since individual response to digitoxin is variable, no clear-cut levels of toxicity are established. The average nontoxic level is about

17 to 20 ng/ml, and toxic is between 26 and 35 ng/ml blood. Radio-immune assay is the method of choice for this drug test. Since this technique is highly specific, the physician must request assay of the drug by name.

Digoxin response is also variable, depending on age and the severity of arterial disease. The threshhold of nontoxic-toxic levels is about 2 ng/ml blood. Radioimmune assay is the method of choice for this drug test, which must be requested by name.

Glutethimide (Doriden)

Toxic level: more than 3 mg/dl

The action of this drug is similar to that of barbiturates. It is poorly soluble in water, and thus gastric lavage is especially useful when overdose is suspected. It is more highly concentrated in adipose tissue.

Hallucinogens

Lysergic acid diethylamide (LSD) and mescalene are the most common drugs in this category. Miniscule doses of LSD produce symptoms, and current methods are not sensitive enough to use for blood or urine screening. The common practice of using sugar cubes as carrying medium makes analysis of these sources of the drug possible.

Metals

Arsenic is a common ingredient of insecticides. Individual sensitivity to the poison appears to depend on the amount and frequency of exposure to insecticides containing arsenic compounds. Sudden onset of nausea, vomiting, and diarrhea are symptoms of acute poisoning. Arsenic appears in the hair in about 30 h after ingestion, and in chronic poisoning, 0.1 to 0.5 mg/100 g hair is possible. In acute poisoning, the levels may reach 3 mg/100 g hair. Urinary excretion of more than 0.1 mg/24 h is considered at the toxic level.

TABLE 4-9   RANGE OF NORMAL VALUES FOR BLOOD CHEMISTRY

(These ranges are a guide to the normal concentrations of
blood constituents. For accurate interpretations, always refer to
normal values established by individual laboratories, since
individual differences in procedures may affect actual ranges.)

Constituent	Range
Aldolase	3–8 Sibley-Lehninger units/dl
Adults	3–8 Sibley-Lehninger units/dl
Children	About 3X adults
Ammonia nitrogen	35–70 μg/dl
Amylase	60–150 Somogyi units
Bilirubin	
Total	0.1–1.2 mg/dl
Direct	0.05–1.4 mg/dl
Indirect	0.4–0.8 mg/dl
Calcium	4.8–5.2 meq/liter
Carbon dioxide	
Content	24–30 mmol/liter
Combining power	50–58 vol/dl
Tension (P_{CO_2})	35–45 mm Hg
Catecholamines	
Epinephrine	0.48–0.51 μg/liter
Norepinephrine	1.55–3.73 μg/liter
Chloride	100–110 meq/liter
Cholesterol	150–250 mg/dl
Cholinesterase	0.5–1.0 pH unit
Copper	
Males	70–140 μg/dl serum
Females	80–155 μg/dl serum
Ceruloplasmin	35–65 IU
Creatine phosphokinase	0–200 sigma units
	0–36 IU
Creatinine	0.5–1.2 mg/dl
Fibrinogen	200–400 mg/dl plasma
Glucose	65–110 mg/dl (Somogyi-Nelson method)
Immunoglobulins	
IgG	800–1,600 mg/dl
IgA	50–250 mg/dl
IgM	40–120 mg/dl
IgD	0.5–3.0 mg/dl
IgE	0.01–0.04 mg/dl

TABLE 4-9 (continued)

Constituent	Range
Iron	
Serum iron	65–170 μg/dl
Total iron-binding capacity	250–400 μg/dl
Lactic dehydrogenase	165–300 units
Lipase (Cherry-Crandall method)	1.0–1.5 units
Lipoproteins	Amounts not used: pherogram patterns given
Magnesium	1.6–2.1 meq/liter
Osmolality	280–290 mOsm/kg
Oxygen	
Content	15–23 vol/dl
Saturation	95–97%
Tension (P_{O_2})	80–90 mm Hg
pH, arterial	7.35–7.45
Phosphatase, acid	1.0–4.0 King-Armstrong units
Phosphatase, alkaline	2.0–5.0 Bodansky units
Phosphorus, inorganic	1.7–2.6 meq/liter
Potassium	4.0–5.4 meq/liter
Proteins (serum)	
Total	6.5–8.0 g/dl
Albumin	4.0–5.5 g/dl
Globulins	
α_1	0.1–0.4 g/dl
α_2	0.4–1.2 g/dl
β	0.5–1.1 g/dl
γ	0.5–1.6 g/dl
Sodium	136–142 meq/liter
Transaminases	
SGOT	10–40 units
SGPT	5–35 units
Triglycerides	10–90 mg/dl
Urea nitrogen (BUN)	8–28 mg/dl
Uric acid	3.0–5.0 mg/dl

Lead is found normally at levels of 0.01 to 0.08 mg/dl blood, with 50 percent in the erythrocytes. Lead combines with sulfhydryl groups of proteins, including enzymes, and produces cellular death. Paint, storage batteries, and unglazed pottery are common sources of lead poisoning. Symptoms vary widely, from anoxia to those simulating brain tumor. Basophilic stippling of the erythrocytes is a common finding. Heparin must be used for the anticoagulant for specimens of blood for lead analysis, since EDTA chelates lead in the same fashion as calcium.

Mercury also combines with sylfhydryl groups of proteins, with the same effect as lead. Potential sources of mercury poisoning include not only mercury compounds and the metal per se, but drugs and fungicides. Trivalent mercury is more dangerous than bivalent mercury. Mercury toxicity develops when there is 30 to 100 μg excreted in the urine per day.

Narcotics

Sensitivity to these drugs is dependent upon individual tolerance levels. They include cocaine, morphine, and methadone. Blood serum is the preferred specimen. Radioimmunoassay is the method of choice for morphine, detecting as little as 25 ng/ml.

REFERENCES

Davidson, Israel, and John B. Henry (eds.): "Todd-Sanford Clinical Diagnosis by Laboratory Methods," 15th ed., Saunders, Philadelphia, 1974.

Faulkner, W. R., J. W. King, and H. C. Damm (eds.): "Handbook of Clinical Laboratory Data," 2d ed., Chemical Rubber Co., Cleveland, 1968.

Filley, Giles F.: "Acid-Base and Blood Gas Regulation," Lea & Febiger, Philadelphia, 1971.

Gonzales, T. A., et al.: "Legal Medicine, Pathology and Toxicology," 2d ed., Appleton-Century-Crofts, New York, 1954.

Hansten, Philip D.: "Drug Interactions," 2d ed., Lea & Febiger, Philadelphia, 1973.

Hoffman, William S.: "The Biochemistry of Clinical Medicine," 3d ed., Year Book Inc., Chicago, 1964.

Metheny, Norman A., and W. D. Snively: "A Fluid Balance Handbook for Nurses," Lippincott, Philadelphia, 1966.

Oser, B. L., (ed.): "Hawk's Practical Physiological Chemistry," 14th ed., McGraw-Hill, New York, 1965.

Page, L. B., and Perry Culver: "Syllabus of Laboratory Examinations in Clinical Diagnosis," rev. ed., Harvard University Press, Cambridge, Mass., 1962.

Searcy, Ronald L.: "Diagnostic Biochemistry," McGraw-Hill, New York, 1969.

Thienes, Clinton H., and Thomas J. Haley: "Clinical Toxicology," 4th ed., Lea & Febiger, Philadelphia, 1964.

Tietz, N. W., (ed.): "Fundamental of Clinical Chemistry," Saunders, Philadelphia, 1970.

Univ. Ill. Hosp. Lab. Bull. (Mimeo.):
    Enzymes, March, 1970.
    Immunoglobulins, April, 1970.
    Lipoproteins, August, 1970.
    Radioimmunoassay, September, 1973.

FIVE

TESTS FOR SPECIFIC FUNCTIONS

In tests for specific functions, the nurse's part in the procedure is quite important to an accurate result. In preparing patients for a test, it is important that they be well-instructed about the procedure so that they can be as much at ease as possible. When the nurse understands the principles and procedures involved in a particular test, she can help patients by informing them about the test and explaining the necessary restrictions that may be involved. She may also have some part in the collection of specimens or supervise those who do this in nursing service. Scheduling is another important part of most tests for specific functions and is often the responsibility of the nurse. Through her understanding and knowledge, she serves the patient and the technologist by helping to ensure optimal cooperation of all concerned.

ENDOCRINE FAMILY

Hormones in Urine

A number of hormones are excreted in the urine, in one form or another. Precise instructions for the collection of 24-h urine specimens are essential for accurate test results. The patient should understand her part in the collection, and the nurse should supply her with proper equipment. The collection of 24-h urine specimens for each of the hormone studies discussed below is done according to the following method:

1. Give the patient a bottle large enough to accommodate the entire specimen.
2. Keep the specimen cold during the collection period in order to inhibit bacterial growth.
3. Caution the patient to collect urine before defecating.
4. Use a preservative according to instructions of the laboratory.
5. Have the patient void at 8 A.M. and discard the specimen.
6. Collect all urine voided between 8 A.M. one day and 8 A.M. the following day, putting each sample in the large bottle provided. Keep it refrigerated all during the collection period.
7. End the collection period by having the patient void at 8 A.M. the day following the beginning of the collection period.
8. Deliver the total specimen to the laboratory as soon as possible after completion of the test period.

Radioimmunoassay

Radioimmunoassay (RIA) may be used to evaluate endocrine-gland status by measuring the amounts of hormones present in the blood serum. It has the advantages of being extremely sensitive and specific. Its sensitivity is shown by the fact that it is possible to measure substances present only in nanograms. The specificity is related to the fact that the technique uses principles of immunology (see Chap. 6). Table 5-1 lists the RIA tests available in endocrine-gland studies and their clinical uses.

TABLE 5-1   RADIOIMMUNOASSAY TESTS AVAILABLE

Material	Used to evaluate
Human growth hormone (HGH)	Pituitary function and growth
Insulin	Diabetes, islet-cell tumors of pancreas
Thyroxine (T_4)	Thyroid function
Tri-iodothyronine (T_3)	Thyroid function
Thyroid-stimulating hormone (TSH)	Pituitary-thyroid axis
Parathormone	Parathyroid function, calcium and phosphate regulation
Adrenocorticotropin (ACTH)	Pituitary-adrenal axis
Cortisol	Adrenal function and corticoid concentration
Follicle-stimulating hormone (FSH)	Pituitary-gonadal axis
Luteinizing hormone (LH)	Pituitary-gonadal axis
Testosterone	Testicular function
Estrogen	Fertility, ovarian function
Progesterone	Ovarian function, pregnancy, fertility
Human placental lactogen (HPL)	Fetal well-being, placental tumors
Aldosterone	Pituitary aldosteronism (adrenal hypertension)
Gastrin	Gastrointestinal disorders

Pituitary Gland

GENERAL CONSIDERATIONS

The pituitary gland might be called the master control center, since its activities affect a wide range of body functions. The *anterior lobe* controls the functions of many of the other endocrine glands through the production of hormones which stimulate action of each specific gland; e.g., thyroid-stimulating hormone, which regulates body growth. The *posterior lobe* secretes vasopressin (blood-pressure control), antidiuretic hormone (water-reabsorption control), and oxytocin (uterine-muscle control). There are no practical laboratory tests available which can measure the levels of pituitary hormones; to assess pituitary capacity, procedures based on the products of the target organs must be used.

In using these procedures, one should understand that there is a delicate mechanism of feedback inhibition involved in the economy of the pituitary. By this is meant the controlling effect of the levels of hormones produced by the target organs. For example, when the levels of thyroxine and tri-iodothyronine are at normally functioning levels, the pituitary production of the thyroid-stimulating hormone, thyrotropin, is shut off. This same process occurs in the other endocrine glands. When body needs require additional specific hormones, or when levels are lower than normal, the pituitary is turned on. Thus, the role of the pituitary gland and its response to feedback is extremely important in the maintenance of general body homeostasis.

Of course, major pituitary dysfunction is also evident in various clinical manifestations, an example being acromegaly seen in adult hyperpituitarism. Differential diagnosis often involves testing pituitary reserves. In these tests, the role of the nurse cannot be over emphasized, since not only must she administer the appropriate drugs at specified times, but she must also make absolutely certain that the specimens required are properly collected.

TESTS OF PITUITARY FUNCTION

Pituitary Reserve

An indirect method of testing for pituitary reserve involves measurement of urinary corticosteroid levels after the patient has received a medication, SU 4885, which inhibits the production of hydrocortisone by the adrenal cortex. As noted above, when normal levels are not present, the pituitary gland responds by producing additional target-organ-stimulating hormone, in this case adrenocorticotropic hormone (ACTH). Under the influence of the additional ACTH, the adrenals secrete higher-than-normal levels of corticosteroids. If the pituitary reserve is limited, there will be no rise in ACTH and no rise in corticosteroid levels. (See pituitary-adrenal-capacity test for interpretation of low adrenal response.) The procedure for the test for pituitary reserve is as follows:

1. A 24-h urine specimen is collected for control, or base-line, determination of corticosteroid level.
2. SU 4885 is given every 4 h for 2 days.
3. The second 24-h urine specimen is collected and corticosteroid level determined.

With normal pituitary reserve, the corticosteroid level of the second urine specimen is two to four times that of the control specimen. If there is impaired pituitary function, no rise in, or an even lower level of, corticosteroid is found.

Corticotropin Suppression

In this test, pituitary-adrenal capacity is involved. Endogenous pituitary ACTH is suppressed by exogenous synthetic cortisol (dexamethasone or Decadron), which is 40 to 100 times as potent as endogenous ACTH and is not part of the urinary metabolites of hormones. The amount of synthetic ACTH required to reduce ACTH levels and, thereby, corticosteroid levels, is dependent upon the state of pituitary activity. The following procedure is employed:

1. A 24-h urine specimen is obtained as a control for base-line ACTH and corticosteroid levels.
2. Synthetic ACTH, 0.05 mg every 6 h, is given over a 2-day period.
3. A second 24-h urine specimen is obtained.

Normally, the ACTH level is reduced by 50 percent or more, and the corticosteroid level falls to 2 mg or less. If a high dose (2 mg) is required, hyperactivity of the pituitary is indicated. This is useful in the diagnosis of Cushing's syndrome.

Adrenal Gland

GENERAL CONSIDERATIONS

From the laboratory standpoint, it is important to understand the distinctions between the various compounds (metabolites of the

TABLE 5-2   NORMAL VALUES OF ADRENAL STEROIDS
AND OTHER HORMONES*

Steroid or hormone	Adult male, μg	Adult female, μg	Children, μg
Corticosteroids (17-keto-genic)	9–22 (decreasing with age)	6–15 (decreasing with age)	Less than 6 (increasing with age to adult levels)
Androgen (17-keto-steroid)	8–18	5–15	3–5
Aldosterone	2–15	2–15	2–15
Catecholamines	8–163	8–163	Not determined
Vanilmandelic acid (VMA) (metabolite of catecholamines)	0.5–7	0.5–7	Not determined

*All values are in terms of 24-h urine excretion.

adrenocortical hormones) which are determined. In the laboratory, the metabolites of cortisol, corticosterone, cortisone, and 11-hydroxycorticosterone are included in the 17-ketogenic, or 17-hydroxysteroids. It should be noted that the term "ketogenic" refers to a laboratory procedure which alters this group of metabolites by their artificial conversion to 17-ketosteroids, since this form is more stable to the processes of analysis. The metabolite of androgen is 17-ketosteroid per se, and no alteration by laboratory means is needed.

The corticoid group of hormones is essential in (1) electrolyte metabolism, (2) water balance, (3) gluconeogenesis, (4) control of protein metabolism, and (5) control of body defense mechanisms. Aldosterone is concerned with electrolyte metabolism.

TEST OF ADRENAL FUNCTION: ADRENOCORTICAL RESERVE

The rationale of this test is based on the response of the adrenal cortex to excess ACTH. The test procedure is as follows:

1. A careful history of previous treatment with ACTH is obtained, since this can result in some degree of adrenal suppression.
2. A control 24-h urine specimen is collected, and corticosteroid level is determined.
3. A specified dose (usually 40 units) of ACTH is given intramuscularly every 12 h for 1 to 3 days.
4. A second 24-h urine specimen is collected for corticosteroid level test.

Normally, the corticosteroid level of the second specimen will be three to four times that of the control specimen. In Cushing's syndrome, the increase reaches ten times that of the control. The control is normal to subnormal in Addison's disease, with no increase in the postmedication specimen. Panhypopituitarism shows a subnormal response.

INDIRECT MEASURES OF ADRENAL FUNCTION

Electrolyte Balance

Sodium. A diagnostic feature in adrenal insufficiency or loss of adrenal tissue is that the serum sodium level is markedly lowered from the normal average of 140 meq/liter. This is largely caused by impaired stimulation of the renal tubular cells to reabsorb sodium when the blood sodium levels are reduced. Loss of sodium via the urine is characteristic of adrenal impairment, particularly as seen in Addison's disease.

Hyperactive adrenal cortex, which is the basis of Cushing's syndrome, produces the opposite effect, and the serum sodium concentration is in the range of high normal (148 meq/liter) to elevated.

As noted in Chap. 4, determination of the sodium concentration in blood is performed on serum, requiring venous blood. There is no need to withhold the diet in preparation for the test.

Potassium. Although there is no consistent rise of the serum potassium level in Addison's disease, it does happen frequently and affects the course of treatment. When it does occur, the potassium level ordinarily does not exceed 7 meq/liter. This is not diagnostic of Addison's disease, since it may occur in a shocklike state with oliguria.

The hyperactive adrenal cortex affects potassium concentration by lowering the level below the low-normal value of 4.0 meq/liter. This is a common finding in Cushing's syndrome.

As noted in Chap. 4, determination of potassium concentration is performed on blood serum, requiring venous blood. There is no need to withhold the diet prior to obtaining the specimen.

Chloride. In Addison's disease, the serum chloride level may be affected; when it is, an elevation is noted. It may reach relatively high levels, and when this occurs, chloride acidosis (which is characteristic of this disease) results. In Cushing's syndrome, the reverse is true, with a tendency toward alkalosis and attendant low chloride levels.

Determination of chloride levels is performed on blood serum. There is no need to withhold the diet prior to obtaining the specimen.

Glucose Metabolism

Hypoglycemia in the fasting state is a common finding in adrenal insufficiency. The glucose level is lower than 80 mg/dl blood. These patients show a marked sensitivity to insulin; the blood glucose level is markedly lowered, and rebound to normal level is slow to occur.

In normal persons, administration of ACTH may raise the blood glucose level beyond the ability of the renal tubules to reabsorb the glucose and thereby produce glycosuria. Patients with diabetes mellitus who are treated with this hormone require more insulin than usual.

Hyperactive adrenal cortex produces hyperglycemia, and in Cushing's syndrome a curve typical of diabetes is seen in glucose-tolerance tests. As one might expect, this condition leads to resistance to insulin. It is noted that patients with diabetes mellitus require much more insulin than their usual dose when they are receiving ACTH.

Since the blood specimen for glucose determination must be

obtained with the patient in the fasting state, breakfast is withheld until the sample is drawn. Venous blood is used for the test.

Water Balance

It has been noted that when a large amount of water is given to a patient with Addison's disease or to one with adrenal insufficiency, diuresis does not occur promptly. On this basis, the Robinson-Kepler-Power test is sometimes used to diagnose this condition.

Preparation of the patient for this test requires that he take no food or fluids after 6 P.M. the evening before the test. The following procedure is then carried out:

1. At 10 P.M., have the patient void and discard the specimen.
2. Save all urine voided thereafter until 7 A.M. and consider it the night specimen. Measure the volume.
3. At 7 A.M., have the patient drink 20 ml water/kg of body weight within 45 min.
4. Collect urine specimens at 8, 9, 10, and 11 A.M. and measure accurately for volume.

If any one of the morning specimens exceeds the total volume of the night specimen, normal adrenal function is indicated. If there is a question whether delayed diuresis might be due to other causes, further evaluation is necessary, based on comparison of the excretion of urea in the night specimen and the blood urea level as determined on a sample of blood drawn the morning of the test. In the normal person, the ratio of urea excreted to blood urea level is significantly greater than 1.

Gonads

ANDROGEN

Normal range (24-h specimen)
Adult male under 60 years: 9–22 mg/24 h
Male over 60 years: gradual decrease due to
reduced testicular activity

In the male, at least a third of the production of androgen is a function of the testes. Testicular androgen appears to have more hormonal potency than that of the adrenal gland. Tests for androgen are useful in evaluating tumors of the testes as well as in diagnosis and treatment of hypofunction or lack of proper development of the testes. This hormone plays a role in the development of secondary sex characteristics.

In adrenogenital syndrome and adrenocortical tumor, there is a marked increase in 17-ketosteroid excretion. Low levels are seen in cases involving hypofunction or lack of proper development of the testes.

ESTROGENS

Normal range (24-h specimen)
Adult male: 4–25 μg/24 h
Adult female: 4–60 μg/24 h (in pregnancy, the level
is about 45 μg)

The essential functions of estrogens (estrone, estradiol, and estriol) are related to the feminizing processes. They are produced in varying amounts by the ovaries, by the adrenals, and, in pregnancy, by the placenta. Determination of urinary estrogen levels can help diagnose malfunction or underdevelopment of the ovaries (although it is not usually necessary to use this test) and certain ovarian tumors. Its most significant use is in diagnosis of ovarian agenesis and ovarian folliculoma.

Elevation of the 24-h estrogen level is seen in adrenocortical tumor, adrenocortical hyperplasia, and some testicular tumors. Low levels are seen in infantilism, ovarian agenesis, Simmond's disease, lutein-cell tumor, and arrhenoblastoma.

PREGNANEDIOL

Normal range (24-h specimen)
Nonpregnant: 0.5–7 mg/24 h
Pregnant: 5.0–15.0 mg/24 h, rising during pregnancy to
47 mg/24 h in the last trimester

When there is threatened abortion due to decreased production of progesterone, the expected rise in pregnanediol concentrations in the urine does not occur. In the presence of corpus luteum cysts, the level may be elevated considerably.

CHORIONIC GONADOTROPIN

Produced by the placenta and by certain tumors, this hormone has a luteinizing effect. It is this hormone which is utilized in various pregnancy tests (Chap. 2).

Parathyroid Glands

Regulation of calcium concentration and absorption is a function of the parathyroid hormone. Impairment or hyperactivity of this gland is evident in the ratio of calcium to phosphate levels. In hyperactivity, the calcium level is elevated, and increased excretion of calcium ions in the urine occurs. In hypoactivity or impaired function, the serum calcium level drops, and an increase in phosphate level is noted, with increased excretion of phosphate in the urine.

Sulkowitch's test for urinary calcium is a simple, roughly quantitative test. The patient is restricted to a low-calcium diet for 3 days before the test. A 24-h urine sample is collected and tested for the presence of calcium ions.

Thyroid

Tests for thyroid function have progressed from the gross assessment of basal metabolic rate (BMR) to measurement of serum iodine, to in vitro and in vivo radionuclide procedures. This progression has been marked by increasing precision in assessing thyroid gland status. The BMR is no longer used; the protein-bound iodine (PBI) and butanol extractable iodine (BEI) have fallen into disuse because of their sensitivity to contamination by extraneous iodine. With the availability of radionuclides of iodine, there is greater precision of measures possible. The first use of ^{131}I was in studies based on iodine uptake, an in vivo test. While this test is very unlikely to cause problems associated with radiation hazards to the patient, it is still desirable to use in vitro tests as much as possible. These tests are now well-developed, the most recent being radioimmunoassay techniques, using ^{125}I or ^{131}I to tag the hormones of the thyroid gland that are bound to serum proteins. With the scintiscans, not only can thyroid uptake of iodine be measured, but it is possible to visualize thyroid tissue and related tumors when present.

As table 5-3 shows, there is a wide variety of physiologic effects that result from the action of thyroid hormones, demonstrating the usefulness of thyroid-function assessment. In Table 5-4, the status of the thyroid gland and types of conditions with which this is associated are shown.

TABLE 5-3   RELATIONSHIPS OF THYROID-RELATED HORMONES

Hormone	Source	Acts on	Influences
Thyrotropin-releasing factor (TRF)	Hypothalamus	Anterior pituitary	Release of formed TSH; synthesis of additional TSH in response to body needs
Thyroid-stimulating hormone (TSH)	Anterior pituitary	Thyroid	Iodine trapping; complexing of iodotyrosines to thyroglobulin; hydrolysis of thyroglobulin; ratio of T_3 and T_4; size and blood supply of thyroid
Tri-iodothyronine (T_3) (all but 0.2% bound to thyroxin-binding globulin)	Thyroid	Selected body systems	Growth and maturation / Cellular oxygen consumption
Thyroxine (T_4) (all but 0.02% bound to TBG and thyroxine-binding pre-albumin)			Anabolism/catabolism / Cardiac rate and output / Sensitivity to epinephrine (blood pressure) / Muscle tone / Glucose absorption / Bone resorption / Enzyme systems

NOTE: Free T_3 (FT_3) is several times more active than FT_4, which balances their quantitative differences.

SOURCE: Based on Israel Davidsohn and John B. Henry (eds.), "Todd-Sanford Clinical Diagnosis by Laboratory Methods," 15th ed., p. 744, W. B. Saunders Company, Philadelphia, 1974.

TABLE 5-4   CONDITIONS REFLECTED BY THYROID STATUS

Thyroid status	Associated conditions
Euthyroidism	Diffuse goiter; uninodular or multinodular goiter; sometimes with benign or malignant tumors of the thyroid; thyroiditis; congenital anomaly
Hypterthyroidism	Diffuse toxic goiter (Grave's disease); uninodular or multinodular toxic goiter; exogenous thyroid hormone; sometimes with benign or malignant tumors of the thyroid
Hypothyroidism	Idiopathic; loss of thyroid mass; iodine deficiency; goitrogens; inborn errors of metabolism; TSH deficiency; TRF deficiency
Decreased thyroid reserve	As noted in hypothyroidism

SOURCE: Based on Israel Davidsohn and John B. Henry (eds.), "Todd-Sanford Clinical Diagnosis by Laboratory Methods," 15th ed., p. 747, W. B. Saunders Company, Philadelphia, 1974.

TRI-IODOTHYRONINE (T_3)

Normal range
    Males: 11–19%
    Females: 11–17%

This test involves incubating the patient's serum with a measured amount of ^{125}I-T_3 or ^{131}I-T_3 and particles of resin, followed by counts of the radioactivity of the serum and the resin. The percent of T_3 that has been adsorbed by the resin is calculated and reported as the result.

TRI-IODOTHYRONINE INDEX (T_3 INDEX)

This test is based on the fact that thyroxine-binding globulin (TBG) has a greater affinity for T_4 than for T_3, and the amount of ^{125}I-T_3 taken up by the serum of the patient is proportional to the number of TBG binding sites not occupies by T_4. Some laboratories use the same materials but count the radioactivity of the resin used to absorb excess ^{125}I-T_3; i.e., they do a T_3RU (T_3-resin uptake) test rather than a T_3SU (T_3-serum uptake) test. T_3RU results are usually reported as percent uptake rather than as an index, and since T_3RU and T_3SU values are inversely proportional, confusion may occur during interpretation. To avoid this, the T_3 index is frequently converted mathematically so that the results are directly proportional.

The T_3 index is calculated by determining the ratio between the unknown T_3SU and the standard euthyroid serum T_3SU. It is necessary to determine the T_4 values in order to interpret the T_3 index.

T_3-INDEX INTERPRETATIONS

Thyroid status	T_3SU index	Corresponding converted value
Euthyroidism	0.92–1.17	0.86–1.09
Hypothyroidism	more than 1.17	less than 0.86
Hyperthyroidism	less than 0.92	more than 1.09

THYROXINE (T_4)

Normal range:
   T_4 iodine: 3.9–7.7 $\mu g/dl$[1]
   T_4:   5.9–11.8 $\mu g/dl$

In this test, ^{125}I-T_4 bound to TBG is used. The ^{125}I-T_4 is displaced by the patient's T_4 proportionately, in equilibrium, and the released radioactive T_4 is measured in percent, which is compared with a standard curve to convert the value to $\mu g/dl$.

FREE THYROXINE INDEX (FTI)

Normal range: 5.7–13.2%

Although more than 99 percent of the T_4 circulating in the blood is bound to TBG or to other serum proteins, it is most likely

[1] T_4-iodine value is calculated by multiplying the T_4 result by 0.653, which is the proportion of iodine present in thyroxine.

TABLE 5-5   INTERPRETATION OF T_3-INDEX AND T_4 RESULTS

T_3-index results	T_4 results	Possible condition
Normal	Normal	Euthyroidism
Elevated	Elevated	Hyperthyroidism
Decreased	Decreased	Hypothyroidism
Elevated*	Decreased*	Nephrosis; TBG deficiency; treatment with androgens, Dilantin, steroids, ACTH; large doses of salicylates or phenylbutazone
Normal*	Decreased*	Hypothyroidism treated with T_3 compounds
Normal	Increased	Any of these findings may be associated
Decreased	Increased	with estrogen therapy, oral con-
Decreased	Normal	traceptives, or pregnancy

*rare
SOURCE: Radioimmunoassay, Univ. Ill. Hosp. Lab. Bull., September, 1973.
(S. T. Nerenberg, M.D., Ph.D., Director.)

that the level of free T_4 actually determines the metabolic status. The ratio of total thyroxine to total available binding sites can be expected to be proportional to the concentration of free thyroxine. The FTI is a measure of this ratio and is calculated by multiplying the T_4 value by the T_3 index. The FTI is normal for euthyroidism regardless of estrogen therapy, oral contraceptives, or pregnancy. The correlation of FTI with clinical disorders is also somewhat better than that with T_3 or T_4 alone.

IODINE UPTAKE

Normal range: 12–35% uptake

This test for thyroid function uses a small dose (5 μCi) of ^{131}I, followed by periodic radioactivity counts of the thyroid gland area after the patient takes the dose; generally the test is completed at 24 h. In order to check on the completion of excretion of the ^{131}I not taken up by the thyroid, the patient collects all urine voided during the test period, and counts are performed to determine the percent excreted.

BERSON ^{131}I CLEARANCE TEST

Normal range:
  Plasma: 8–10 ml cleared/min
  Urine: 30–40 ml cleared/min

In this test, 24 μCi ^{131}I is given to the patient intravenously, and the ^{131}I count of the thyroid area is recorded continuously for 30 min. Urine is collected at the end of the test period. The results of the test are most commonly reported in numbers of milliliters of plasma cleared of ^{131}I per minute by the thyroid gland. In making the calculations, it is necessary to account for the "iodide space" of the body, which is related to body weight. The iodine is accounted for in terms of that which is diffused into the body generally, that which is excreted in the urine, and that which is trapped in the thyroid gland. Since exogenous iodine in the blood and tissues (not related to thyroid hormones) can distort the values, it is also important to have information on the patient's diet and the possibility of his having taken proprietary drugs containing iodine.

Specific instructions will be provided for preparation of the patient and procedures required during testing periods for both the uptake and the Berson clearance tests.

GASTRIC ANALYSIS

General Considerations

Analysis of gastric contents for acidity and volume can be an important aid to the diagnosis of benign ulcers and pernicious anemia. Interpretation of gastric-analysis results must be made in the light of other findings, including radiographic examinations and clinical history. In pernicious anemia, the results of gastric analysis are somewhat like screening-test results and must be followed by more definitive tests.

Elevated gastric acidity is common with benign ulcers. It is less definitive in differential diagnosis of other gastric problems. Achlorhydria, confirmed by lack of response to stimulation with histamine or preferably, Histalog, is characteristic finding in untreated pernicious anemia.

Preparation of the Patient

All gastric analyses require that the patient be in the fasting state. She may not smoke the morning of the test until the test is completed, since smoking stimulates the gastric mucosal secretory cells. Extraneous stimulation is to be avoided so that the test will be under controlled conditions. In the alcohol, caffeine, and histamine methods, it might be well to inform the patient that the test will require the passing of a tube into her stomach, although in some cases such warning might make it more difficult for her to help, as she must, with the process. Anticipation of this particular process can increase her discomfort. Admittedly, it is an unpleasant experience, however necessary it may be.

Gross Appearance of Gastric Aspirate

Bile, indicated by yellowish to greenish discoloration, is not normally found unless the patient retches or gags during passage of the tube to the stomach. Marked amounts of bile usually indicate the need to investigate the possibility of obstruction high in the intestinal tract.

Mucus is a normal constituent of gastric aspirates. Gastric mucus is miscible with the fluid, and oral mucus appears as globs floating on the surface of the specimen. Mucus from the upper respiratory tract is tenacious and frequently contains particles of pigment.

Blood in small amounts may result from trauma associated with passage of the tube or with too-vigorous suction in removing the specimen from the stomach. If aspiration of bloody material other than in streaks occurs, the tube must be removed immediately.

Determination of Acidity

Gastric-juice acidity is a combination of electrolytes, weak un-ionized acids, and hydrochloric acid. Modern methods of measuring gastric acidity are based on pH determinations with the glass electrode, converting this value to milliequivalents of hydrogen per liter using the Moore-Scarlata nomogram.

TABLE 5-6   AVERAGE FINDINGS IN GASTRIC ACIDITY AND VOLUME

Condition	Normal		Duodenal ulcer	
	Acidity, meq/liter	Volume, ml/h	Acidity, meq/liter	Volume, ml/h
Fasting	2.5	62	5.6	85
30 min after Histalog stimulation	10.5	110	17.0	154

STIMULANTS FOR GASTRIC-ACID PRODUCTION

Alcohol

In this method, 50 ml of 7% ethyl alcohol is given to stimulate gastric activity. The test requires about 1½ h and is done in the following manner:

1. Give the patient no food after her evening meal the night before the test is to be done. She may have water during the evening but nothing by mouth on the morning of the test.
2. Pass the Levin tube to the patient's stomach and aspirate the gastric contents.
3. Introduce 50 ml of 7% alcohol into the stomach through the Levin tube.
4. Obtain specimens of the gastric contents at 15- to 20-min intervals up to 1 h.

Caffeine

Roth and Ivy devised this method of studying gastric activity. A solution of 0.5 g caffeine sodium benzoate in 2 dl water is used as the stimulating agent. Specimens of gastric secretion are then aspirated at 30-min intervals up to 2 h after the meal. This meal is particularly of value in diagnosing duodenal ulcer, as the results show a greater secretion of acid in a shorter period of time than in normal subjects or in patients with other types of disease.

The test requires about 2½ h, and the test procedure is as follows:

1. Give the patient no food after her evening meal the night before the test is to be done. She may have water during the evening but nothing by mouth on the morning of the test.
2. Pass the Levin tube to the patient's stomach and aspirate the gastric contents.
3. Introduce a solution of 0.5 g caffeine sodium benzoate in 2 dl water into the stomach through the Levin tube. Note time.
4. Obtain specimens of gastric contents 30 min after the test meal and every 10 min thereafter up to 2 h.

Histamine

Histamine has been found to be a potent stimulus to gastric secretion. It is convenient to use, and the gastric contents are easily aspirated. Histamine must be used with great care, since severe allergic responses may result in the sensitive person. For this reason, Histalog (histamine analog) is to be preferred, for it gives comparable results in stimulation with much lower incidence of reaction. When histamine is used, it is important to perform a skin test to determine the patient's possible sensitivity to histamine. Lack of response after stimulation with histamine is diagnostic of pernicious anemia in those cases in which hematologic findings indicate the possibility of such disease. In cases in which the diagnosis in question is benign peptic ulcer, lack of response to histamine is considered by most gastroenterologists to rule out this condition.

This test requires about 1½ h, and the procedure is as follows:

1. Give the patient no food after her evening meal the night before the test is to be done. She may have water during the

evening but nothing by mouth on the morning of the test.
2. Inject 0.1 ml histamine diphosphate intradermally. The test is positive if the wheal and erythema exceed 10 mm in diameter. A positive result indicates that the patient is hypersensitive to histamine, and its use is contraindicated.
3. Pass the Levin tube to the patient's stomach, and aspirate the gastric contents.
4. Administer 0.01 mg histamine diphosphate/kg body weight *or* 0.5 mg Histalog/kg body weight intramuscularly.
5. Obtain specimens of gastric contents at 15- to 20-min intervals up to 1 h.

Note: Side effects of histamine (and to a lesser extent, Histalog) must be watched for. These include flushing of the face, headache, and possibly a drop in the blood pressure. *Histamine is not to be given to patients with history of asthma, urticaria, and other allergic conditions.*

DIAGNEX BLUE TEST

All other methods of gastric analysis require aspiration of gastric contents. In the Diagnex methods, free hydrochloric acid is tested by indirect, qualitative means. Free hydrochloric acid releases a dye, azure A, from a resin base. The dye (indicator) is absorbed by the gastrointestinal tract and excreted in the urine. The urine is then tested for the presence of the indicator. The obvious advantage of this method is that it does not subject the patient to the discomfort of having a Levin tube passed into his stomach. It is a valuable screening test, since positive results indicate secretion of hydrochloric acid, which may be sufficient information for the diagnosis. However, in those cases in which hydrochloric acid is not secreted, further investigation with the use of histamine or Histalog is indicated before a conclusive result can be obtained.

The Diagnex Blue test requires 2 h, and the procedure is as follows:

1. Give the patient no food after her evening meal the night before the test is to be done. She may have water during

the evening and on the morning of the test.
2. Have the patient void at 8 A.M. and save the specimen.
3. Give the patient a capsule containing caffeine. Mix the packet of dye resin with a glass of water and give it to the patient 1 h after taking the caffeine. An additional glass of water may be taken. Note the time.
4. Have the patient void again 1 h after taking the dye resin and save the specimen.
5. Take the two urine specimens to the laboratory for analysis.

KIDNEYS

Tests for Active Renal Lesions

This group of tests gives an indication of the degree of pathologic process that may be present but does not yield information about physiologic aspects of function. The group includes tests for urinary protein, blood pigment in the urine, blood cells (both red blood cells and white blood cells) in the urine, and casts in the urine.

URINARY PROTEIN

Proteinuria is a consistent finding in nephrosis and nephritis; most cases show a marked proteinuria. Although quantitative determinations of protein in urine may be made in these cases, they do not necessarily indicate the state of the disease process. In nephritis, quiescence brings rapid decrease in the proteinuria. Persistent proteinuria of a severe degree leads to the nephrotic state. The tests for proteinuria have been discussed in Chap. 2.

BLOOD PIGMENT

When erythrocytes break down, the hemoglobin is released into the medium in which the cells are found. The term used to indicate the presence of hemoglobin in the urine is "hemoglobinuria." In acute nephritis, many red blood cells pass through the damaged walls of the glomerular capillaries, and hemoglobinuria is a consistent finding in this disease. The partial disintegration of the red blood cells leads to hemoglobinuria, and this, with the presence of red blood cells, gives the smoky appearance to such urine. Hemoglobinuria is seen in cases of severe chemical intoxications and after hemolytic transfusion reactions, blackwater fever, and paroxysmal nocturnal hemoglobinuria.

BLOOD CELLS

As would be expected, any infectious process in the urinary tract is accompanied by the presence of leukocytes in the urine, the severity of the infection being indicated by the number of cells observed in microscopic examination of the urine.

Red blood cells may be present in the urine in a variety of diseases, It is important to know the source of the bleeding to make a definitive diagnosis. When the bleeding is located in the kidneys, there is a tendency toward formation of red blood cell casts and development of hemoglobinuria. When the bleeding is from the lower urinary tract, no such casts are seen, of course. Frank blood may be present, or blood may be revealed only by microscopic examination.

CASTS

Casts are molds of the renal tubules and are formed when protein in the urine precipitates within the tubules. They are present in serious renal disease and are accompanied by proteinuria. Casts containing white blood cells and/or red blood cells may be seen. Sloughed epithelial cells may also be incorporated into casts. When these various cells disintegrate within the cast, it becomes a granular in appearance. Noncellular casts are hyaline in appearance. The presence of casts in the urine is an indication of possible renal lesions and further investigation should be made.

Tests for Renal Functional Capacity

This group of tests includes those which measure the ability of the kidneys to rid the body of a foreign substance (dyes), to concentrate the urine, to function in maintaining electrolyte and water balance, and to excrete products such as urea, which are removed from the body in the urine.

PHENOLSULFONPHTHALEIN TEST

Abbreviation: PSP
Normal range: 40–60% excretion, first hour; an
additional 20–25%, second hour
Time required: 2 h

Although more accurate means of obtaining information about renal function are available, this test is still fairly common. It gives limited information because rather marked kidney damage must be present before the test gives significantly abnormal results. The procedure is as follows:

1. The patient may have a light breakfast and one glass of water, but no coffee or tea.
2. Inject 1 ml (0.6 mg) phenolsulfonphthalein, preferably intravenously, and *note the exact time.*
3. Give the patient one glass of water to drink.
4. Collect a urine specimen 15 min after injection of the dye.
5. Give the patient another glass of water.
6. Collect urine specimens 1 and 2 h after injection of the dye.

Note: When the dye is given intramuscularly, collect the urine specimens 1 h 10 min and 2 h 10 min after the injection.

FISHBERG'S CONCENTRATION TEST

A simple method of determining renal function is to test the ability of the kidneys to produce concentrated urine. A good indicator is the specific gravity of a random sample of urine: if the specific gravity is 1.018 or greater, it may be assumed that the kidneys are functioning within normal limits.

This test requires that the patient have no food or water from the evening meal the night before the test is to be done until after completion of the test period (11 A.M.).

1. Give the patient dinner at 6 P.M. or earlier.
2. No food or water may be taken until completion of test period.
3. Collect urine specimens at 10 and 11 A.M. the following morning.
4. Test the urine specimens for specific gravity.

In normal concentration, the specimens will have a specific gravity of 1.020 or greater. In the absence of diabetes insipidus, specific gravity lower than 1.020 indicates impairment of renal function.

ELECTROLYTE AND FLUID BALANCE

Essential to electrolyte balance is the function of the kidneys in filtering and reabsorbing or excreting electrolytes as part of the urine. Factors that impair filtration will lead to retention, and those which impair normal reabsorption will lead to loss of electrolytes. Extrarenal conditions have a profound influence on both these procedures. For example, in Addison's disease there is marked loss of sodium due to the inability of the kidneys to respond to the necessity of conserving sodium, which is secondary to lack of adreno-corticotropic hormone. As pointed out above, obligatory reabsorption of water and electrolytes occurs in the tubular portion of the nephron unit, so that almost 90% of the water in glomerular filtrate is reabsorbed, carrying along with it sodium, chloride, bicarbonate, phosphate, potassium, calcium, and magnesium in amounts similar to those in glomerular filtrate. Disturbances in the electrolyte and water balances can, therefore, result from impaired or absent extrarenal stimuli, which are provided by the hormones governing these functions. Dehydration and hyponatremia are also seen in diseases marked by fluid loss through severe vomiting or diarrhea.

With an intrinsic kidney disease such as uremia, the damage to the nephron unit is direct and obviously impairs its efficiency. Here again, filtration and reabsorption are affected, but from a mechanical cause: cellular damage. The effects of loss of water, sodium, and chloride, as well as the other manifestations of disease, result in renal damage if untreated, and the patient is caught in a vicious circle of ever-increasing seriousness.

Tests for the electrolytes (sodium, potassium, chloride, and bicarbonate) are performed on blood serum and thus require venous blood. Any of the substances may be tested for at any time during the day; thus it is not absolutely necessary that the patient be in the fasting state. For further discussion of these substances, see Chap. 4.

CLEARANCE TESTS

Strictly speaking, "clearance" means complete removal of one substance from another medium. For example, 30 students in a room each have 1 pencil; if the teacher collects these 30 pencils, he has "cleared" the students of pencils. In renal function, clearance of a substance from the blood is accomplished by filtration and excretion. Thus, with the discovery of substances that are primarily subject to filtration in the glomerulus, glomerular function can be assessed. By the same token, those substances which are primarily subject to excretion by renal tubules afford a valuable tool in assessing tubular mass and tubular function.

Urea

Time required: 3 h
Range of normal: 60–90 ml/min (average clearance: 75 ml/min)

An obvious choice for study of renal function is urea, because it is an excretory product of the kidney. However, since not *all* the plasma flowing through the kidneys is filtered and since a portion of the urea that is excreted is reabsorbed, the term clearance can be applied only in a relative sense. Nevertheless, this is a valuable test in evaluating renal function.

The patient is given his regular breakfast, and he may smoke during the test. He may be up and about, provided he understands about the collection of urine specimens at specified times.

1. At 7 A.M., give the patient breakfast with plenty of fluid.
2. At 7:30 A.M., give the patient two glasses of water to drink.
3. At 8 A.M., have the patient empty his bladder completely and discard the sample.

4. At 9 A.M., have the patient empty his bladder completely again and save the entire amount. *Note the exact time in minutes.*
5. Draw a blood sample for urea nitrogen determination.
6. At 10 A.M., have the patient empty his bladder completely again and save the entire specimen.
7. Draw a blood sample for urea nitrogen determination.

Urea nitrogen determinations are made on the urine and blood samples, and the amount of blood cleared of urea per minute is calculated.

Inulin

Average rate: 130 ml blood/min

Since inulin, a polysaccharide, is not reabsorbed by the renal tubules, it can be used to determine the effectiveness of the glomeruli, yielding information regarding glomerular filtration rates (the amount of blood filtered per minute). The test is not done routinely, however, and requires special equipment in the laboratory.

TUBULAR FUNCTION

Average rate: 77 mg/min

Substances (Diodrast, hippuric acid, and aminohippuric acid) have been discovered that are excreted by the renal tubules, thus affording a method of assessing tubular function. p-Aminohippuric acid (PAH) is a compound in common use for this purpose. By determining blood and urinary p-aminohippuric acid levels at a specified time after injection of the compound, the maximal tubular excretory capacity for PAH is found. This is called Tm_{PAH}. Tm indicates the maximal about of reabsorption that occurs. Since the tubules are able to reabsorb limited amounts of certain substances, different substances have different normal Tm's. Like the inulin clearance test, this determination is not done routinely because it requires special equipment not available in the average laboratory.

LIVER

As may be expected from the wide variety of vital processes accomplished by the liver, tests of its functional integrity involve an equally wide variety of determinations. These tests are classified according to function: *excretory, metabolic,* and *detoxicating.* In addition, there is a group of tests based upon alterations in serum protein patterns.

TABLE 5-7 THE NORMAL HEPATOGRAM

Function	Test	Normal range
Excretory	Bromsulfalein	With 2 mg/kg dose, less than 4% retention at 30 min
	Alkaline phosphatase	2–4 Bodansky units
	Bilirubin	Direct: 0.0–0.2 mg/dl
		Total: 0.2–1.4 mg/dl
	Icterus index	8 units or less
	Urobilinogen	Trace
	Cholesterol	Total: 135–260 mg/dl
		Ester: 95–200 mg/dl
	Cholinesterase	0.7–1.4 pH units/h
	Lactic acid dehydrogenase	Less than 300 units
	Transaminase (SGPT)	5–35 units
	Serum proteins	Total: 6.5–8.0 g/dl
		Albumin: 4.0–5.5 g/dl
		Globulin: 2.0–3.0 g/dl
		Fibrinogen: 0.2–0.3 g/dl
	Prothrombin time	12–15 s
	Prothrombin production	Shortening of prothrombin time after dose of vitamin K
Metabolic	Galactose tolerance	Oral: less than 3 g excreted in 4 h
		Intravenous: complete removal 45–60 min
Detoxication	Hippuric acid	Oral: at least 3 g excreted in 4 h
		Intravenous: at least 1 g excreted in 1 h
Miscellaneous	Cephalin flocculation	Negative to 2+
	Zinc turbidity	4–8 units
	Thymol turbidity	1–4 units

Excretory Function

ALKALINE PHOSPHATASE

Normal range: 2–4 Bodansky units

Although the mechanism that causes increased alkaline phosphatase in obstructive jaundice is not fully understood, tests for the increase are useful in differential diagnosis of liver disease with jaundice. Alkaline phosphatase is excreted in the bile, and it is thought that in obstructive jaundice the alkaline phosphatase is returned to the bloodstream with the bile, thus producing an elevated level. In obstructive jaundice, the level is more than 10 units. In viral hepatitis there may be some elevation, but the level is not more than 10 units. The alkaline phosphatase isoenzyme in liver is type 1.

BILIRUBIN

Bilirubin production is related to hemoglobin breakdown. Normally, about 7.5 g hemoglobin is reduced every 24 h. This produces 35 mg bilirubin/g hemoglobin, or a total of 260 mg/day. All but 1 percent of this bilirubin is excreted in the feces, after alteration to urobilinogen and urobilin by action of intestinal-tract bacteria. The remaining 1 percent is excreted in the urine as urobilinogen.

Free bilirubin (indirect form) is unconjugated and is bound to plasma protein, chiefly to albumin. It is not soluble in water and hence cannot be excreted in the urine. It is the major contributor to the clinical signs of jaundice. *Conjugated bilirubin* (direct form) is bilirubin which, through the action of the liver, has glucuronic acid or sulfate attached to the basic structure of its molecule. It is water-soluble, and therefore it can be excreted in the urine unaltered.

The characteristic pathologic findings in various types of jaundice are as follows:

1. Obstructive jaundice
   a.   Increased free bilirubin in plasma
   b.   Decreased fecal urobilinogen

      c.   Decreased urine urobilinogen
      d.   Increased urine bilirubin
2. Defective conjugation by the liver
      a.   Increased free bilirubin in plasma
      b.   Decreased urobilinogen
      c.   No urine bilirubin
3. Overproduction of bilirubin (e.g., hemolytic anemia)
      a.   Increased free bilirubin in plasma
      b.   Increased fecal urobilinogen and urobilin
      c.   Increased urine urobilinogen
      d.   No urine bilirubin
4. Hepatocellular jaundice
      a.   Increased free bilirubin in plasma
      b.   Normal-to-decreased fecal urobilinogen
      c.   Increased urine urobilinogen
      d.   Bilirubin in the urine

With the use of Ictotest[1] for detecting small amounts of bilirubin in the urine, a valuable aid to diagnosis is available, since it has been found that there can be positive urine bilirubin without any suspicion of liver disease—it precedes the obvious appearance of the symptoms. It is recommended that this test be made one of the routine procedures of urinalysis.

Two methods are used in testing for urobilinogen in the urine. One gives the report in terms of Ehrlich units, and the other as a titer. An Ehrlich unit is specified as that equivalent to one milligram pure urobilinogen per deciliter of solvent. Less use is being made of 24-h determinations for urobilinogen, which have been supplanted by the 2-h afternoon collection of urine. This is because it has been found that maximal excretion of urobilinogen occurs in midafternoon to early evening. The nurse's responsibility in this test is to be sure to note the total time during which collection was made and to make sure that the total specimen is sent to the laboratory, since the volume of specimen is critical in determining the result. As with any determination for urobilinogen, the specimen

---

[1] Ictotest is the product of the Ames Company, Elkhart, Ind.

TABLE 5-8   DIFFERENTIAL DIAGNOSIS OF MEDICAL
AND SURGICAL JAUNDICE

Tests	Medical		Surgical	
	Uncomplicated	Obstructive	Uncomplicated	With cholangitis
Urine uro-bilinogen	Elevated	Lowered	Lowered	Elevated
Cephalin floccu-lation	4+	4+	Negative	Negative
Alkaline phos-phatase	Less than 15 Bodansky units	Less than 15 Bodansky units	More than 15 Bodansky units	More than 15 Bodansky units
Cholesterol	Normal to low	Normal to low	Elevated	Elevated
% of choles-terol esters	Marked decrease	Marked decrease	Normal	Normal
SGOT	Marked elevation	Marked elevation	Slight elevation	Slight elevation
Prothrom-bin time, with vita-min K	Impaired	Impaired	Normal	Normal
Stool color	Brown	Clay	Clay	Clay
Liver biopsy	Parenchymal disease	Parenchymal disease, with bile stasis	Bile stasis	Bile stasis with cholangitis

SOURCE: After L. B. Page and P. J. Culver, "Syllabus of Laboratory Examinations in Clinical Diagnosis," Harvard University Press, Cambridge, Mass., 1960, by permission of the publisher.

should be taken to the laboratory without delay. This is necessary because bacteria which may be present in the urine act upon urobilinogen, oxidizing it to urobilin.

BROMSULFALEIN

Abbreviation: BSP

This tests the ability of the liver parenchymal cells to remove a dye introduced into the circulatory system. The rate of removal is influenced by hepatic blood flow, the functioning capacity of the polygonal cells, and the freedom of the biliary tract from obstruction.

The test requires the patient to be in the fasting state. About 1½ h is required for the test. Three venipunctures will be done. Ordinarily there is no reaction to injection of the dye, but the patient should be observed for any allergic type of reaction.

1. The patient is to be in the fasting state.
2. Obtain blood by venipuncture for control sample.
3. Slowly give Bromsulphalein (2 mg/kg body weight) intravenously. Note the time when the injection is completed.
4. Obtain blood by venipuncture 30 min and 1 h after the injection. Take it from the opposite arm.

Normally there is less than 5-percent retention of the dye 1 h after the injection. An elevation above this level would indicate liver damage.

CHOLESTEROL, CHOLESTEROL ESTERS

The liver plays an important role in both the synthesis and the excretion of cholesterol. Cholesterol is excreted in the bile and is the free form. As expected, obstructive jaundice produces an elevation of the serum cholesterol level. When the liver cells are damaged, the ester fraction of the total cholesterol level is decreased, and the total cholesterol level is at about the normal level.

CHOLINESTERASE

It has been noted that the cholinesterase level is decreased in hepatitis, and the test may be used to aid in differential diagnoses of jaundice, since the cholinesterase level is unchanged in obstructive jaundice.

TRANSAMINASES

Since the liver is one of the organs rich in transaminases (particularly glutamic-pyruvic transaminase), this test is an important diagnostic aid in evaluating degrees of liver damage due to hepatitis. Of the two transaminases, glutamic-oxaloacetic and glutamic-pyruvic, the latter is found in greater amounts in the liver.

LACTIC ACID DEHYDROGENASE

While not ordinarily used as part of the study of liver disease, it is important to remember that this enzyme (LDH-1) is present in rather large amounts in liver tissue, and thus the LDH could be elevated in liver damage. In the differential diagnosis of myocardial infarction, this is an important point.

SERUM PROTEINS

Because the liver plays a large role in the synthesis of proteins that are part of the normal composition of blood, alterations in the amounts of these proteins (albumin, globulin, fibrinogen) may be expected in diseases of the liver parenchyma, with lowered levels or alteration of the ratio of the proteins to each other resulting.

PROTHROMBIN TIME

The liver synthesizes prothrombin, an important factor in coagulation of the blood. When the liver is seriously damaged, the prothrombin time is prolonged because of inadequate production by the liver.

PROTHROMBIN PRODUCTION

This tests the response of the liver to a dose of vitamin K, as reflected by the prothrombin time. It is determined by checking the prothrombin time before, and 24 h after, injection of 2 mg vitamin K. The normal response to this dosage is a shortened prothrombin time, compared with that obtained before.

Metabolic Function

GALACTOSE TOLERANCE

Galactose is a sugar which is absorbed from the intestinal tract intact and which is converted to glycogen by the liver. Consequently, within certain limits the rate of disappearance of galactose reflects the health of the liver. Two methods of performing the test are in use: in one, galactose is administered orally; in the other, intravenously. The latter method is considered to be more accurate because it is not affected by the rate of absorption from the intestinal tract.

The oral test requires 5 h to complete, during which time the patient eats nothing. He may have water ad lib. Urine specimens are used for analysis.

The procedure in the oral method is as follows:

1. The patient is to be in the fasting state.
2. Give the patient a solution of 40 g galactose in 4 dl water. Note the time when this is taken.
3. Collect urine specimens *each hour* for 5 h.

If more than 3 g galactose are excreted in the 5 h, liver damage is preventing conversion of galactose to glycogen.

The intravenous method requires about 2 h to complete, and since the determinations for galactose are performed with blood, at least two, and possibly six, venipunctures are necessary. The procedure is as follows:

1. The patient is to be in the fasting state.
2. Give galactose (0.5 g/kg body weight) intravenously. Note the time when the injection is completed.
3. Draw blood 15 and 45 min after injection. (For a complete curve, samples are drawn every 15 min for 90 min.)

At 15 min the blood galactose level should be between 100 and 200 mg/dl and at 45 min there should be no galactose present if the liver is functioning normally. The galactose-removal constant normally lies between 4.2 and 9.5 percent/min. In hepatic disease, it is about 1.5 percent.

Detoxication Function

HIPPURIC ACID TEST

Although the kidneys can convert benzoic acid to hippuric acid, this conversion is performed chiefly by the liver. Hippuric acid is normally present in the urine in concentrations up to 0.7 g/24 h. In the hippuric acid test of liver function, a precise dose of sodium benzoate (a salt of the acid) is given, and the urine is analyzed for the amount of hippuric acid excreted in a given period of time after the dose. Pathologic impairment of hepatic function is indicated by decreased hippuric acid excretion. The intravenous method is preferable to the oral because it is independent of the rate of absorption from the intestinal tract and can be completed in less time.

The oral method requires 4 h to complete. The patient need not necessarily be in the fasting state. The procedure is as follows:

1. Give the patient a solution of 6 g sodium benzoate in 2.5 dl water. Note the time.
2. Collect all urine voided in the 4 h after ingestion of the dose, and analyze it for hippuric acid.

Excretion of less than 2.5 g hippuric acid indicates liver damage. The intravenous method requires 1 h to complete according to the following procedure:

1. Have the patient empty his bladder completely.
2. Give the patient a glass of water.
3. Slowly give 1.77 g sodium benzoate in 20 ml distilled water intravenously, over a period of 5 to 10 min. Note the time when injection is completed.

4. Collect a urine specimen 1 h after the injection was completed, and analyze it for hippuric acid.

Excretion of less than 0.7 g hippuric acid indicates liver damage.

Miscellaneous Tests

This category includes tests based upon alterations in serum proteins. The alteration of protein concentration and structure leads to easy precipitation of the γ-globulin fraction and to a coagulative effect on colloidal suspension. In all these tests, it is necessary to collect blood with the patient in the fasting state.

THYMOL TURBIDITY

Normal range: 1–4 units
Source of blood: Venipuncture

Upon the addition of serum to an aqueous solution of thymol, the γ-globulin precipitates, giving the solution a turbid or cloudy appearance. The degree of turbidity depends on the concentration of γ-globulin, which may be increased when the liver is damaged.

ZINC TURBIDITY

Normal range: 4–8 units
Source of blood: Venipuncture

Like the thymol turbidity test, this is a rough measure of the γ-globulin concentration.

PANCREAS

Tests of pancreatic function are concerned with pancreatic secretions: the enzymes *amylase, lipase,* and *trypsin.* Of course, since it is the site of the production of insulin, disease states related to this important substance will be reflected in the metabolism of carbohydrates.

Examination of Aspirate

The hormone secretin stimulates the secretion of pancreatic digestive juices, which contain the enzymes. This is used to test pancreatic activity. The pancreatic juice is aspirated from the duodenum after an injection of secretin, and the material is tested for volume and amount of the various enzymes present. Impaired function of the pancreas is reflected in reduced volume and in low enzyme concentrations.

As in the case of aspiration of gastric contents, the patient may experience some discomfort from having the tube passed. In testing pancreatic function, a special tube with two openings, one for the stomach and the other for the duodenum, is necessary. This tube is used so that gastric secretions will not be mixed with those of the pancreas. It may be necessary to check the position of the tube to the duodenum fluoroscopically, which entails a minor radiologic procedure.

Examination of Stool

Examination of the stool also affords a good indication of the state of pancreatic function. When the pancreas is functioning improperly, the stools are bulky, pale in color, of a greasy, putty-like consistency, and have a rancid odor.

The tests for amylase and lipase are discussed in Chap. 4. It is noted here that the amount of both these enzymes is increased in acute pancreatitis.

Trypsin is tested for by a simple qualitative method devised by Schwachman. This test is primarily of value in infants and children. It is performed on a specimen of stool which must be relatively soft. Trypsin deteriorates during a delayed passage through the colon, and therefore a specimen of constipated stool might yield erroneous results.

Sweat Tests

In cystic fibrosis of the pancreas, important diagnostic tests are based on the alterations found in the electrolyte composition of sweat, notably in the marked increase of chloride excretion. Screening tests which are used include the fingerprint test (modified Webb test) or handprint test (modified Schwachman test). When a positive screening test is obtained, a more precise diagnostic test must be performed—either the thermal sweat test or iontophoretic sweat test. In the former, sweating is induced by increasing body temperature. In iontophoretic tests, sweating is induced by electrical introduction of pilocarpine in a small area.

FINGERPRINT TEST

The Webb fingerprint tests uses as the indicator medium a small filter paper impregnated with a combination of 2 percent silver nitrate and 10 percent potassium chromate. The patient is instructed to rub the thumb and forefinger together to stimulate sweat production, and then holds the impregnated paper firmly for 5 s. A positive result is indicated by a color change in the reagent from brownish-red to bright yellow. Duplicate positive tests should be obtained before results are regarded as significant. A follow-up diagnostic test must be performed to confirm the screening-test results.

HANDPRINT TEST

The modified Schwachman test utilizes agar or impregnated filter paper containing silver chromate and is based on precipitation of silver chloride in the presence of sweat containing chloride in excess of 50 meq/liter. A finger, hand, or toe imprint is made on the test medium after washing the part to remove possible chemical contaminants. When there is little chloride on the skin surface, the imprint is barely detectable, but in the presence of increased chloride content, a clear, white to yellowish print is seen, caused by the precipitation of silver chloride.

IONTOPHORETIC SWEAT TEST

In iontophoresis, a low level of electric current is applied to the test area (usually the volar surface of the forearm) through gauze containing pilocarpine hydrochloride. Pilocarpine is a sudorific alkaloid, and its introduction by iontophoresis induces sweating in the exposed area. After this initial treatment, the sweat is collected on filter paper and analyzed for chloride content in relation to the amount of sweat obtained. Values of 50 meq/liter or more are diagnostic.

PULMONARY-FUNCTION TESTS

While these tests are not performed by the laboratory's personnel, it is pertinent to discuss them as part of this section on specific functions.

Pulmonary-function tests find their greatest use in (1) clinical study and classification of chronic lung disease, such as emphysema, bronchitis, and asthma, (2) the evaluation of therapy and prognosis in chronic lung disease, (3) the preoperative evaluation of patients needing resectional surgery, (4) the determination of pulmonary disability, and (5) the evaluation of the breathless patient.

Ventilation Tests

Ventilation tests measure the ability of the patient to fill and empty the lungs. These tests are expressed in liters or in liters per unit time (for the rapid tests). Values are also expressed in terms of percent of the predicted normal, based on expected values for a given age, sex, and height. Reliable ventilation tests are usually performed with spirometers. The following are the ventilation tests:

1. The vital capacity is a measure, in liters, of the amount of air that the patient can expel from completely inflated lungs. This is a measure of that part of the lung which is available for ventilation.
2. The timed, forced expiratory volume (FEV) measures the amount of air that can be forced out of fully inflated lungs in a given time. Usually, the FEV-0.75 sec, FEV-1 sec, and FEV-3 sec are

measured. The FEV is dependent on the vital capacity and the patency of the airways. The FEV is expressed in liters per unit time or in percent of vital capacity. For example, the FEV-1 sec is normally at least 75 percent of the vital capacity.

3. The maximum midexpiratory flow (MMEF) measures air expelled in liters per second during the middle portion of a forced expiration. This test is independent of airway patency and is the most sensitive index of obstruction to air flow.

4. The maximum breathing capacity (MBC), or maximum voluntary ventilation (MVV), measures the total ability of the patient to move air in and out of the lungs. This test is dependent on open airways, vital capacity, muscle strength and effort, coordination, and the enthusiasm of the technician conducting the test. It is very reproducible if properly performed, and probably remains the single most useful ventilation test.

Diffusion Tests

These tests measure the uptake of carbon monoxide across the alveolar-capillary membrane. With loss of the alveolar-capillary membrane, as in emphysema, or in diseases causing thickening of the membrane, such as in fibrosis, carbon monoxide uptake is impaired. These tests can be performed at rest or with exercise. They are most reliable when performed with exercise.

Lung Volumes and Compartments

The total lung volume (TLV) or total lung capacity (TLC) measures the size of the lungs and dead space in liters. The residual volume (RV) is a measurement, in liters, of the air which cannot voluntarily be expressed from the lungs. The TLV and RV are measured by rebreathing an indicator gas such as helium. The RV can be determined by measuring the nitrogen "washed out" of the lungs while breathing pure oxygen. Total lung volumes and residual volumes increase in emphysema. By contrast, in bronchitis the RV is increased, but the TLV is normal or nearly so.

Blood Gas Analysis

The ultimate function of the cardiorespiratory system is to adequately oxygenate the blood and maintain a normal concentration of carbon dioxide. Measurement of arterial pH, oxygen and carbon dioxide partial pressures, and hemoglobin saturation indicates the overall ability of the lungs to maintain normal blood gas function.

TABLE 5-9   PULMONARY TESTS IN ASSESSMENT
OF RESPIRATORY FAILURE

Defect	Refelction of abnormality
Ventilation	
1. Obstructive a. Emphysema b. Bronchitis c. Asthma d. Strangulation	1. Decreased MBC, FEV-1 sec, MMEF. In asthma, these results are reversible in part with bronchodilator drugs
2. Restrictive a. Fibrosis b. Kyphoscoliosis c. Pleural thickening d. Obesity	2. Some decrease in MBC; nearly normal FEV-1 sec, MMEF
3. Neuromuscular impairment a. Poliomyelitis b. Curarelike drugs	3. Decreased MBC and VC
4. Lack of respiratory drive	4. Decreased MBC and VC
Gas Exchange	
1. Pulmonary fibrosis granulomas a. Sarcoidosis b. Hamman-Rich syndrome c. Berylosis	1. Decreased diffusion of carbon monoxide; often, decreased oxygen partial pressure and oxygenation of hemoglobin
2. Severe emphysema	2. Decrease in all measures of diffusion and gas analysis
3. Pulmonary edema	3. Decreased oxygen partial pressure and hemoglobin oxygenation
4. Chronic obliterative pulmonary vascular disease	4. Decreased carbon monoxide diffusion, oxygen partial pressure, and hemoglobin oxygenation
5. Anatomical loss of functioning lung a. Pleural effusion b. Massive pneumothorax	5. Decreased carbon monoxide diffusion, oxygen partial pressure, and hemoglobin oxygenation

REFERENCES

Dale, Sidney: "Principles of Steroid Analysis," Lea & Febiger, Philadelphia, 1967.

Davidsohn, Israel, and John B. Henry (eds.): "Todd-Sanford Clinical Diagnosis by Laboratory Methods," 15th ed., Saunders, Philadelphia, 1974.

Fishberg, A. M.: "Hypertension and Nephritis," Lea & Febiger, Philadelphia, 1954.

Freeman, J. A. and M. F. Beeler: "Laboratory Medicine—Clinical Microscopy," Lea & Febiger, Philadelphia, 1974.

Hamolsky, Milton: "Thyroid Testing," Lea & Febiger, Philadelphia, 1970.

Hoffman, William S.: "The Biochemistry of Clinical Medicine," 3d ed., Year Book, Chicago, 1964.

Oser, B. L. (ed.): "Hawk's Practical Physiological Chemistry," 14th ed., McGraw-Hill, New York, 1965.

Radioimmunoassay, Univ. Ill. Hosp. Lab. Bull., (mimeo.), September, 1973.

Searcy, Ronald L.: "Diagnostic Biochemistry," McGraw-Hill, New York, 1969.

Tietz, N. W. (ed.): "Fundamentals of Clinical Chemistry," Saunders, Philadelphia, 1970.

SIX

IMMUNOLOGIC EXAMINATIONS

GENERAL CONSIDERATIONS

Serology is the study of immune bodies, which are the direct product of the defense mechanisms against disease processes. In the late nineteenth century, studies of immunologic phenomena were begun systematically and intensively. Although the practice of vaccination had been common for over a century, the relationship between causative agents and the body's defense mechanisms was not pursued until the attention of Pasteur, Ehrlich, Koch, Wasserman, and others was drawn to this field. With the development of methods for isolating disease-causing organisms, Koch and others were able to demonstrate the basis of infectious diseases, and Koch's classic postulates came to be accepted.

All the concepts of immunology are built upon two elements:

188

antigen and *antibody*. An antigen is a substance, usually protein in nature, which, upon inoculation in a susceptible animal, incites the development of a corresponding substance, the purpose of which is to neutralize the antigen or render it susceptible to the body's natural defenses. This latter substance, which is manufactured in response to an invading foreign substance, is called an antibody. Antibodies are characterized by the way in which they are demonstrated serologically. They include (1) agglutinins, (2) precipitins, (3) complement-fixing antibodies, (4) hemagglutinins, (5) hemolysins, (6) cytolysins, (7) opsonins, (8) neutralizing antibodies, and (9) hemagglutinin inhibitors.

Antibodies are found in the γ-globulin fraction of serum proteins. Within this group, five classes have been identified: IgG, IgM, IgA, IgD, and IgE. The Ig is the abbreviation for immunoglobulin. These classes are identified by sedimentation constant, molecular weight, peptide chains, carbohydrate fraction, and immunoelectrophoresis. Immunoelectrophoresis is a process combining separation of proteins by electrophoresis and antigen-antibody precipitation. About 80 percent of the antibodies synthesized in response to bacterias, viruses, and toxins are of the IgG class. Cells which contribute to antibody formation include lymphocytes and plasmacytes and lymphoid fixed-tissue cells. Suppression of antibody formation is of primary concern in organ transplants and autoimmune diseases. The agents which have been used for this purpose include chemical agents and drugs, radiation, steroid hormones, and antilymphocyte serum. Chemical agents and drugs interfere with synthesis of antibodies. Radiation destroys tissue. The mechanisms of steroid immunosuppression have not been fully elucidated. Use of antilymphocyte serum obviously is based on immunologic processes.

Immunoglobulin	*Activity*
IgG	Antibacterial, antiviral
IgA	Antibody in external secretions
IgM	Initial response to new antigens, antipolysaccharide
IgE	Reaginic antibody
IgD	Unknown

Radioimmunoassay Tests (RIA)

Radioimmunoassay combines use of principles of immunity and biochemistry and incorporates use of radionuclides such as ^{125}I, ^{131}I, ^{14}C, and ^{3}H. The radionuclides make it possible to detect minute amounts of test materials. The two outstanding characteristics of RIA are its great sensitivity and specificity. Physiologic substances can be measured in nanograms (10^{-9} g) or picograms (10^{-12} g) per milliliter ranges. This degree of sensitivity is essential for determining levels of constituents present in the serum in minute amounts. The RIA specificity is due to the fact that it is based on the antigen-antibody reaction, a highly specific immuno-chemical reaction. A third important characteristic of RIA is its relative validity, or accuracy, compared to biochemical (bioassay) procedures.

Fluorescent-antibody Test

Coons and Kaplan developed a method of coupling fluorescein dye with antibodies and then coating the substance under investigation with this material. After excess antibody is washed off, the substance is examined under the fluorescent microscope. This is a valuable tool in localizing the site of an antigen and in visualizing very small amounts of antigen. It may be used with a variety of substances from bacteria to red blood cells.

In studies of bacterial diseases, it is used to determine, without time-consuming culture techniques, the type of organism causing the disease. It is used to determine the presence of coating or blocking antibodies in Rh and related studies of red blood cells and is extremely useful in this connection.

SEROLOGIC DIAGNOSES

Bacterial Infections

Serologic studies are important aids in diagnosing many bacterial diseases. The ease with which antigens may be prepared from pure cultures of organisms facilitates this procedure. The usual test is the agglutination test. Complement fixation is sometimes used, although it is not usually necessary. The principle underlying the *agglutination test* is that antibodies present in the serum of the patient with a given bacterial disease will cause a suspension of killed organisms of that disease to clump, with the degree of clumping related to the concentration of antibodies present.

The diseases most frequently tested for by agglutination tests are the bacillary dysenteries, tularemia, and brucellosis (undulant fever). Agglutination tests are also used to identify organisms isolated from patients with bacterial diseases, especially the dysenteries.

In rheumatic fever, the common serologic test used is a hemolysin test, the anti-streptolysin O test (ASTO). Streptolysin O is a substance elaborated by streptococci against blood cells.

Agglutination and precipitation tests are reported in terms of the dilution of the serum that will still demonstrate the presence of antibody, expressed as titer. For example, a positive reaction with typhoid organisms at a dilution of 1 part of serum to 39 parts of diluent would be expressed as "positive, 1:40," or "titer 1:40."

Virus Infections

In addition to culturing for specific viruses, viral diseases can be diagnosed by one of the serologic tests. In virus infections, two specimens of serum from the patient are necessary in order to have firm evidence of the particular disease suspected: one taken during the acute phase and one during the convalescent phase. They are necessary to establish whether there has been a rise in titer during the illness, since, in most virus infections, the antibody titers are not of very great magnitude. Consequently, a rise in titer is more significant than the actual titer. A threefold rise in considered diagnostic. The two samples of serum are tested at the same time so that conditions influencing the titers will be the same, thus avoiding technical error. Of the serologic tests used, the complement-fixation, hemagglutination-inhibition, and neutralizing-antibody tests are most important.

COMPLEMENT FIXATION

Complement-fixation tests are based on the fact that complement, a normal protein substance found in all animals and in man, is essential to any antigen-antibody reaction. When complement is used up in this reaction, it is said to be *fixed*, and a subsequent test applied to the serum yields no reaction. In the complement-fixing phase of the test, the antigen used is the organism of the suspected disease.

HEMAGGLUTINATION

Many viruses cause development of agglutinins, which clump red blood cells when the serum of the unknown is reacted with chicken red blood cells treated with the known virus. This is the hemagglutination antibody.

HEMAGGLUTINATION INHIBITION

Influenza

In 1941, Hirst discovered that serum of persons who had influenza prevented the agglutination of chicken red blood cells which ordinarily clumped when treated with the virus of influenza. Inhibition of the hemagglutination phenomenon is used as a serologic means to diagnose the type of influenza.

Rubella

A variation of this type of test is used to determine immunity to rubella. Rubella is a mild febrile exanthema of short duration in children and adults. Its seriousness is as a potential danger to the fetus if the mother contracts the disease during the early months of pregnancy. Fetal infection may occur, with damaging effects on fetal growth and development. Tests for rubella are used to detect hemagglutinin-inhibition antibodies. Detection of any antibodies in the mother's serum is deemed sufficient to protect the fetus, *if* the antibodies are present before pregnancy.

Problems in interpretation usually arise from timing with respect to specimen collection and clinical symptoms. Hemagglutinin-inhibition antibodies in response to natural rubella infection reach a relatively high level quickly and tend to remain so for as long as 10 years. First appearance of the antibodies occurs within 3 days of the onset of rash or 17 days after exposure. When it is not known whether the patient has a previously established antibody titer, it is advisable to obtain a second specimen and test it along with the original. A fourfold rise in titer is indicative of active disease. The usual titer is between 1:32 and 1:64.

NEUTRALIZING ANTIBODY

It has been noted that immune serum (i.e., serum from an animal that has recovered from a specific disease) will prevent the development of that virus in the chick embryo. The test is used much less frequently in clinical practice than are the other serologic tests, because it is more involved and more expensive, but it is a valuable research tool for determining new species of viruses.

Syphilis

The abbreviation frequently used for requesting any of the tests for syphilis is *STS*. Specific tests for this disease are named for the person who devised the test. Two types of tests are done in the standard laboratory: flocculation tests and complement-fixation tests. The *Treponema pallidum*-immobilization (TPI) test must be done in a special laboratory. Fluorescent-treponemal-antibody (FTA) tests require special equipment not ordinarily maintained by a routine laboratory and thus must also be done by a laboratory specializing in this procedure.

Unlike the majority of antigen-antibody tests which make up serology, the standard tests for syphilis are not based on specific antigen derived form *T. pallidum*, the organism causing syphilis. This imposes certain limitations on the tests, but they are nevertheless valuable and reasonably accurate, the accuracy being enhanced by adequate history and clinical findings. The antibody, reagin, is present in the serum of syphilitic persons within a few weeks after infection. The nature of reagin is not completely known. Reagin may also be noted in the serum of some individuals who do not have syphilis. The response of reagin production has been seen in leprosy, tuberculosis, infectious mononucleosis, malaria, collagen diseases, and a few virus infections. When the patient obviously has not been exposed to syphilis but has a positive reaction to one of the serologic tests for syphilis and a negative reaction to TPI or FTA, the reaction is termed a biologic false positive (BFP). It is always advisable, in the presence of a BFP, to investigate further along the lines suggested by the other diseases known to produce such a reaction.

FLOCCULATION

Names of tests: Kline, Kahn, VDRL

These tests are based upon the fact that antigen-antibody reactions result in flocculation, or precipitation, of appropriate parts of the test ingredients. The antigen is originally an emulsion, but upon exposure to its particular antibody, the emulsion is dispersed and the particles of antigen separate out to a degree depending upon the amount of antibody present. Flocculation tests for syphilis are much easier to perform than complement-fixation tests are, but they are less specific and so are used as screening procedures. A positive flocculation test is confirmed by a complement-fixation test on the same serum. By far the most common flocculation test used in the VDRL, which gets its name from the laboratory that perfected it: the Venereal Disease Research Laboratory of the United States Public Health Service.

Rapid screening tests that are used when large numbers of subjects are to be tested, as in a field survey, are the PlasmaCriT (PCT) and the Rapid Plasma Reagin (RPR) tests. They are useful because they allow large-scale testing in a short period of time and with a minimum of equipment. However, they are *only* screening tests. Any positively reacting specimen must be tested by one of the more specific procedures.

COMPLEMENT FIXATION

Names of tests: Wassermann, Kolmer, Reiter

As mentioned in the section on tests for viruses, complement is a protein substance normally present in the serum of animals and man. It is essential to the antigen-antibody reaction. Its consumption in an invisible reaction is tested indirectly by a visible reaction such as hemolysis. When complement is used up, it is fixed in the reaction; hence the descriptive name for this type of test.

A modification of the Kolmer complement-fixation test uses an antigen derived from the treponemal spirochete causing disease in rabbits. The antigen is the Reiter protein. Since the antigen is obtained from organisms related to the organism causing disease in humans, it is considered to be more specific than other antigens commonly used.

Treponema pallidum IMMOBILIZATION

The most sensitive and specific test for syphilis is the TPI, in which the serum is mixed with a sample of live organisms that cause syphilis. The organisms are observed for loss of mobility due to the action of the specific antibody for that organism. It is especially useful in determining the validity of other tests for syphilis, since they can give false positive results (so-called biologic positive). In connection with this test, it is becoming more frequent practice to determine the amount of complement that is fixed in this particular reaction. Such a test is called the *T. pallidum* complement-fixation test (TPCF).

FLUORESCENT-ANTIBODY TEST

Developed from techniques devised by Coons in labeling antibodies with fluorescent dye, the fluorescent-antibody test was produced in 1957 by Deacon and his coworkers. The FTA is less demanding technically and less expensive but still requires special equipment. The antigen used is made up of killed *T. pallidum* organisms. Modifications of Deacon's procedure have made this test highly specific, but it is less sensitive than the TPI, particularly in late syphilis.

Rickettsial Infections

It is of interest to note that, in certain rickettsial diseases, the nonpathogenic organism *Proteus* OX-19 is agglutinated by serum of persons with these diseases. This test is used particularly in presumptive diagnosis of Rocky Mountain spotted fever and typhus and is sometimes known as the "Weil-Felix reaction." More specific tests must be done to confirm such a diagnosis serologically but a presumptive diagnosis of these diseases may be made when there is a fourfold rise in the titer of specimens collected during the acute and convalescent phases of the disease. Complement-fixation and agglutination tests are used in rickettsial diseases.

Mycotic Infections

Systemic, or deep, fungous diseases are diagnosed, in part, by use of the complement-fixation test. It is used quite extensively in the diagnosis of histoplasmosis, a disease caused by the fungus *Histoplasma capsulatum*. This disease affects the lungs, and since it may radiologically simulate miliary tuberculosis in its acute stage, it is important to distinguish between these two diseases in order that proper treatment be given.

Infectious Mononucleosis

Although the causative organism of infectious mononucleosis has not been conclusively isolated, it is commonly thought to be viral in nature. The diagnosis of this disease is confirmed by a positive heterophile agglutination test.

"Heterophile" is defined as "having an affinity for more than one group or species." In this connection, heterophile refers to the sheep red blood cells used in this test. Normally man does not have an antibody against sheep red blood cells, but certain conditions elaborate an antibody that cuases sheep red blood cells to clump. Disease conditions that show a heterophilic antibody are serum sickness and infectious mononucleosis. In infectious mononucleosis, the heterophile antibody is present in titers ranging from 1:56 to as much as 1:2,028. A titer of 1:56 is considered diagnostic.

Primary Atypical Pneumonia

Two tests are of value in confirming diagnosis of primary atypical pneumonia: the cold hemagglutinin and the streptococcus-MG antibody.

COLD HEMAGGLUTININ

In about 50 percent of cases of primary atypical pneumonia, an antibody is elaborated that causes clumping of the patient's own or type O human blood cells at refrigerator temperatures. This is often called the "cold agglutinin test," but it is more precise to label it the "cold hemagglutinin test." Because the word "cold" is part of the name, the test is often incorrectly thought by the uninformed to have a relationship with the common cold.

ANTI-STREPTOCOCCUS MG

Streptococcus MG is not ordinarily a pathogen, but it has been isolated from many cases of primary atypical pneumonia, and in these cases an antibody is developed against this organism. Like the cold hemagglutination test, the streptococcus-MG-antibody test is not uniformly positive in pneumonias of this type. The antibody causes clumping (agglutination) of the organisms.

Rheumatoid Arthritis (RA)

Patients with rheumatoid arthritis may develop a heterogenous group of IgM to form the rheumatoid factor (RF). RF-antibody tests are based on agglutination of either sensitized sheep red blood cells or latex particles coated with an IgG fraction. These tests vary in specificity and sensitivity, and results also vary in relation to the stage of the disease. Most clear-cut titers are seen in advanced disease. Positive results are obtained in about 60 percent of cases of early disease. Titers of 1:80 or higher are considered diagnostic. Screening tests are available, but these are more sensitive than specific and require follow-up titer testing and clinical findings to evaluate positives.

The C-reactive-protein-agglutination test is also used to diagnose and evaluate rheumatoid arthritis (see next section).

Antinuclear Antibody (ANA)

Although a number of tests have been developed for use in assessing tissue-antigen antibodies, the most useful and well-established is the ANA for diagnosis of systemic lupus erythematosus. In contrast with other tests for LE, the ANA is positive in more than 95 percent of the cases. It is a fluorescent-antibody test.

C-REACTIVE PROTEIN (CRPA)

This test is used to diagnose and evaluate inflammatory diseases (particularly rheumatoid arthritis and myocardial infarct) and active, widespread malignant disease. Tissue necrosis and inflammation give rise to the C protein. The C protein is a somatic polysaccharide of the pneumococcus. A similar substance is present in the blood and body fluids of patients with bacterial infections and noninfectious inflammatory diseases. When the C protein and specific antiserum for it are mixed, a fine line of precipitation of the protein occurs This precipitation is graded in degrees from 1+ to 4+.

CARCINOEMBRYONIC-ANTIGEN ASSAY (CEA)

The primary use of the CEA test is as an aid in monitoring treatment of colorectal or pancreatic carcinoma. It is an RIA procedure. There is no fixed pattern of values lending themselves to specificity and sensitivity in diagnosis, since wide variations of values in normal, nonmalignant disease and in malignancies have been found. Generally speaking, in the absence of disease, patients (except for smokers) have levels of 2.5 ng/ml or less. CEA assays are most useful when followed in serial determinations. Extirpation of malignant tumors is marked by a reduction in the CEA level. Persistent increases in CEA levels have been associated with lack of response to treatment or recurrence of disease. In some cases, an elevation occurred several months prior to clinical symptoms. The test is delicate, complicated, and expensive; therefore, it must be used judiciously and always in conjunction with other tests and clinical findings.

IMMUNOLOGY IN TISSUE TRANSPLANTS

The development of equipment permitting extracorporeal circulation and of surgical techniques required for tissue or whole-organ transplants have given the "open sesame" to dramatic means of treating diseases. However, the problems met in these developments were simple compared to those of tissue rejection. The complexity of tissue rejection is complicated by the subtleties of immunologic phenomena, the need for precision in pretesting donor and recipient for possible incompatibilities, and the fact that the immune reaction is so thoroughly a matter of individual differences. There is yet to be found a means of immunosuppression which does not completely rob the patient of capacities to respond to the threats to his life by everyday antagonists—capacities which are taken for granted because they function so imperceptibly and so powerfully that we are seldom aware of them.

Tissue typing to match donor and recipient is dependent upon (a) the nature of the antigen, (b) route of administration, (c) responsiveness of the recipient, and (d) possible preformed antibodies in the recipient. Each of these is well-defined in the classic and long-used procedure of blood transfusion. Although this procedure is common, it is by no means simple, for each of the factors mentioned has to be accounted for and precautions must be taken. In other types of tissue transplant, an additional factor, cell-bound antibodies, must be taken into consideration, for these antibodies are the primary source of graft rejection.

Preparation for transplants involves matching of the blood groups and subtypes, detection of leukocyte and platelet antibodies, determination of lipoprotein type, and, ideally, specific tissue typing. An ideal histocompatibility test is the in vivo skin graft from donor to recipient. However, this has distinct disadvantages in that it requires considerable time and can readily trigger heightened immune response when the desired organ is transplanted. To avoid development of the immune response in the recipient by direct trial, one might think that using a third individual as a walking incubator to test compatibility would be a possibility, but in practice such a procedure is too fraught with risk for the third individual, is expensive, and does not provide sure enough grounds for interpretation.

The normal lymphocyte test, in which recipient lymphocytes are injected intradermally into the prospective donor, has been used. There are disadvantages in this test too, such as the risk of hepatitis and the lack of specificity, since the response in the donor may not be solely due to lymphocytes. Culture of donor and recipient lymphocytes together shows a high rate of blastogenesis in incompatibilities, but it is not possible to identify the source (donor or recipient) of the cells showing this unless the donor cells are treated with mitomycin C. This test requires 7 days for completion and defies quantitation, but it holds promise of usefulness.

Many human leukocyte groups have been serologically identified. Human leukocyte antigens 1, 2, 3, 5, 7, 8, 9, 10, 11, 12, and 13 are tested for in the antiserum panel, using recipient and donor sera. Matching is guided by the detection of similarities between donor and recipient patterns. An abbreviated hypothetical example is seen in Table 6-1.

TABLE 6-1   HUMAN LEUKOCYTE-ANTIGEN
PANEL RESULTS

Serum	HLA			
	1	2	3	5
Recipient*	4+	0	4+	3+
Donor A	0	4+	2+	0
Donor B	4+	0	4+	2+
Donor C	2+	0	0	3+

*Donor B is most likely to match.

Obviously, before the drama of organ transplant can be matched with long-term success in prolonging life with minimal risks, much more needs to be learned about the mechanisms of tissue rejection and immunosuppression, and techniques will have to be developed to answer the nagging questions posed by the inherent problems.

REFERENCES

Bodily, H. L., E. L. Updike, and J. O. Mason (eds.): "Diagnostic Procedures for Bacterial, Mycotic, and Parasitic Infections," 5th ed., American Public Health Association, New York, 1970.

Davidsohn, Israel, and John B. Henry (eds.): "Todd-Sanford Clinical Diagnosis by Laboratory Methods," 15th ed., Saunders, Philadelphia, 1974.

Dubos, Rene J. (ed.): "Bacterial and Mycotic Infections of Man," 4th ed., Lippincott, Philadelphia, 1965.

Eisen, H. N.: "Immunology, An Introduction to Molecular and Cellular Principles of the Immune Response," Harper & Row, New York, 1974.

Fudenberg, H. H., J. R. Pink, D. P. Stiles, and A. C. Wang: "Basic Immunogenetics," Oxford, New York, 1972.

Gray, David F.: "Immunology, an Outline of Basic Principles," American Elsevier, New York, 1970.

Horsfall, F. L., Jr. (ed.): "Viral and Rickettsial Infections of Man," 4th ed., Lippincott, Philadelphia, 1965.

Humphrey, J. H., and R. B. White: "Immunology for Students of Medicine," 3d ed., Davis, Philadelphia, 1970.

Krugman, S., and R. A. Ward: "Infectious Diseases of Children," 4th ed., Mosby, St. Louis, 1968.

Lennette, L. H.: "Diagnostic Procedures for Viral and Rickettsial Diseases," 3d ed., American Public Health Association, New York, 1965.

Manual for Serologic Tests for Syphilis," *Public Health Publ. 411,* 1969.

Parker, C. W.: Radioimmunoassays, in M. Stephaine (ed.), "Progress in Clinical Pathology," Chap. 2, Grune & Stratton, New York, 1972.

Radioimmunoassay, *Univ. Ill. Hosp. Lab. Bull.* (mimeo.), September, 1973.

Skelley, D. S., et al.: Radioimmunoassay, *Clin. Chem.,* **19**:146, 1973.

SEVEN

IMMUNOHEMATOLOGY

All its name indicates, this field of laboratory medicine is concerned with the antigens and antibodies of the blood cells. Since study of the red blood cell antigens and antibodies has a longer history and since methods for their detection are firmly established, it is natural that immunohematology is associated primarily with red blood cells. Another reinforcing factor in this understanding is the fact that the majority of the functions of the blood bank have been focused on transfusion services in the treatment of red cell loss or reduction of blood volume.

Expansion of the field is a natural consequence of advances in immunology technology, of need for services to support advances in the treatment of patients with coagulopathies, and of selection of histocompatible donors for organ transplants. Immunologic studies of platelets and white blood cells have not only proved useful clinically but offer explanations of some previously unidentified complications of transfusion therapy.

Immunohematologic studies contribute to the understanding of the intricacies of genetics. It has been predicted that information provided by immunohematology will lead to increased knowledge about locations and incidence of genes that make up chromosomes; such is knowledge that can be applied to solving non-hematologic-related problems.

The critical importance of transfusion services is attested to by the fact that in 1974, a federal law was enacted to establish a national blood policy commission. In part, this is the result of recognition that existing regulations on biologic products was inadequate to deal with the concerns associated with transfusion and related services.

HISTORY AND NOMENCLATURE OF BLOOD GROUPS

The major blood groups A, B, and O were discovered by Landsteiner in 1900, group AB being discovered in 1902 by van Decastello and Sturli. The antibodies to these blood groups were thought at first to be naturally occurring (i.e., not induced by exposure to antigen), since persons with blood group A cells had antibodies to group B cells; whereas group B cells were accompanied by anti-A antibodies, and group O cells by both anti-A and anti-B antibodies. Subsequent investigations showed that substances chemically similar to A and B antigens are found in plant and animal food source, and this explained the incidence of anti-A and/or anti-B antibodies in the absence of exposure to an incompatible blood group antigen. These group-specific substances are complex mucopolysaccharides containing glucosamine and galactosamine. Blood-group-A- and B-specific substances are found in red blood cells, platelets, white blood cells, and tissues of the exocrine glands such as the pancreas, salivery glands, and those of the gastric mucosa. Blood-group-A-specific substance is derived from porcine gastric mucosa, and group-B-specific substance from equine gastric mucosa for commercially prepared products. Antibodies to groups A

TABLE 7-1   COMPARISON OF BLOOD GROUP ANTIBODIES

Anti-A, anti-B	γ-Globulin type	Placental transfer	In vitro hemolysis	Neutralization by blood-group-specific substances
Natural (Isoagglutinins)	A, B: IgM O: IgG/IgM	Neg	Rare	Complete
Immune*	IgG	Pos	Common	Incomplete

*Developed in response to exposure to the antigen.

SOURCE: Adapted from Israel Davidsohn and John B. Henry (eds.), "Todd-Sanford Clinical Diagnosis by Laboratory Methods," p. 381, W. B. Saunders Company, Philadelphia, 1974.

and B antigens are isoagglutinins.

Four subgroups of A have been identified: A_1, A_2, A_3, and A_X. Among people with the A antigen, which includes group A and group AB types, 78 percent are subtype A_1, 22 percent are A_2, a rare individual is A_3, and an extremely rare person is A_X.

In 1939, Levine and Stetson described a case of maternal-fetal blood incompatibility resulting in hemolytic disease in the infant. This was explained the following year when Landsteiner and Wiener reported discovery of the Rh factor. They named the factor "Rh" because they had used rhesus monkeys in their research. Subsequent research has revealed not a single Rh factor but six, with several variants of these basic factors. Rh_0 (D in the Fisher-Race nomenclature) is highest in incidence and also most antigenic. When an individual's cells contain Rh_0, the term "Rh positive" applies. Rh-negative individuals do not have this antigen; these people are symbolized as Hr_0, or d. Other Rh factors are rh′ (or C) and rh″ (or E); corresponding absences of these factors are hr′ (or c) and hr″ (or d). The Rh factors occur as genetically controlled elements in combination; e.g., one might have a genotype of Rh_0/rh′/hr′ (DCe in the Fisher-Race nomenclature). True Rh-negative individuals have the genotype Hr/hr′/hr″ (cde).

In work by various immunohematologists over a period of years beginning in 1927, when Landsteiner and Levine reported discovery of the M and N factors, a second set of blood factors was recognized. This is the MNS system, which includes a number of different antigens. Antibodies to these factors may occur naturally or as a result of sensitization. They are not highly antigenic and thus are not usually a cause for concern in hemolytic reactions. Other red cell antigen systems have been identified. In the 13 independent and best-defined systems, there are 50 factors which are of practical importance in terms of transfusion service. The MNS, Kell, Duffy, Kidd, P, and Lewis systems are the most frequently included in the panel of cells used in investigation of immunohematology problems. The MNS system may be useful in medicolegal problems involving disputed parentage. The H antigen, a polysaccharide, is found most commonly in association with group O types. It is considered a precursor substrate for group A and group B substances.

In all, more than 200 factors have been identified so that the potential for more than a million different phenotypes exists. Thus, it may be possible to identify individuals by blood-factor patterns as characteristic as fingerprints.

HOW BLOOD TYPES ARE DETERMINED

Blood types (factors) are inherited characteristics and demonstrate the laws of genetics. The individual may be homozygous

TABLE 7-2 NAMES AND SYMBOLS OF SELECTED BLOOD SYSTEMS

System	Symbol	Symbols of factors
Rh-hr	Rh-Hr	Rh_0, rh', rh'', Hr_0, hr', hr'' (Wiener nomenclature)
		D C E d c e (Fisher-Race nomenclature)
Kell	K	K1, K2, K3, K4, K5
Duffy	Fy	Fy^a, Fy^b, Fy
Sutter	Js	Js^a, Js^b
Lewis	Le	Le^a, Le^b
Kidd	Jk	Jk, Jk^a, Jk^b
P		P_1, P_2, p, p^k
Lutheran	Lu	Lu^a, Lu^b, Lu
Xg	Xg	Xg^a (Xg^b is postulated)

(i.e., have inherited the same gene from each parent) or heterozygous (have inherited different genes from each parent). The genotype demonstrates this principle, as shown in Table 7-3, which identifies the genes inherited from each parent, called the genotype. Phenotypes are the expression of genes and thus are observable. Linkage is related to characteristics found in several succeeding generations governed by genes on the same chromosome. For example, factor Xg^a is common to females and thus is sex-linked. There are no tests for identification of genes themselves, but they can be identified by their expression, i.e., the effect they have. When they are expressed only in homozygous and not in heterozygous cells, the genes are termed recessive. When one gene but not the other is expressed in the heterozygous cells, that gene is termed dominant. In codominance, there is equal expression of the genes, e.g., AB blood type.

The general terms for the factor contained in the red blood cells is agglutinogen, since the antigen stimulates the production of agglutinating antibodies. Thus, when red blood cells with a

TABLE 7-3   BLOOD TYPES OF PARENTS AND POSSIBLE
BLOOD TYPES OF OFFSPRING

Parental genotypes	Corresponding parental phenotypes	Possible phenotypes of offspring	Impossible phenotypes of offspring
O/O + O/O	(O + O)	O	A, B, AB
O/O + O/A	(O + A)	O, A	B, AB
O/O + A/A	(O + A)	A	B, AB, O
O/O + O/B	(O + B)	O, B	A, AB, O
A/O + B/O	(A + B)	A, B, AB, O	None
A/O + A/O	(A + A)	A, O	B, AB
A/A + A/A	(A + A)	A	AB, B, O
A/A + B/O	(A + B)	A, AB	O, B
A/A + B/B	(A + B)	AB	A, B, O
O/O + A/B	(O + AB)	A, B	O, AB
A/O + A/B	(A + AB)	A, AB, B	O
A/A + A/B	(A + AB)	A, AB	B, O
B/B + A/B	(B + AB)	B, AB	A, O
A/B + A/B	(AB + AB)	A, B, AB	O

given agglutinogen (factor) come in contact with the agglutinin specific for it, the result is agglutination, or clumping, of the cells. Hemolysis may also be associated with the antigen-antibody reaction.

These two elements, agglutinogen and agglutinin, are the foundation of blood typing. In normal circumstances, antibodies are not produced if the antigen is present in the cells. In the ABO system, the agglutinins are naturally present, as described above. These facts permit determination of these blood types without the individual's having been exposed to the antigen through transfusion of an incompatible type of blood, for example. An additional advantage in ABO typing is the fact that the antigen-antibody reaction occurs at a wider range of thermal conditions; whereas others require a temperature of 37°C for the reaction.

To determine the ABO blood type, the technologist mixes a saline suspension of the unknown red blood cells with each of two antisera: anti-A and anti-B. These sera are the knowns of the equation. For example, if the cells contain group A agglutinogen, the mixture with anti-A serum will show clumping and that with anti-B serum will not. Reverse typing, in which unknown serum is mixed with known cells, may also be done. In the other blood systems, which do not have naturally occurring antibodies, identification is made by using known anti-serum for the factor in question. Figure 7-1 shows the blood-typing reactions in the ABO and Rh systems.

LEUKOCYTE AND PLATELET ANTIGENS

Leukocyte

Two series of leukocyte antigens have been identified; they are distinguished by the terms A and four. In series A, the first to be identified, the genes have been found at locus A on the chromosome. In the second series, series four, the genes are at locus four on the chromosome. There have been 105 phenotypes identified in the A series; 78 in the four series. Combining the two, there are 8,190 possible phenotypes. Applying knowledge of genetics, it is expected

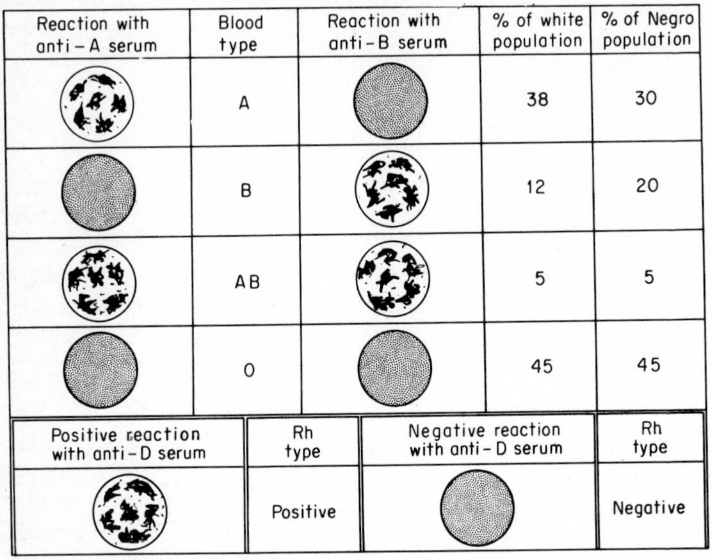

Reaction with anti – A serum	Blood type	Reaction with anti – B serum	% of white population	% of Negro population
	A		38	30
	B		12	20
	A B		5	5
	O		45	45

Positive reaction with anti – D serum	Rh type	Negative reaction with anti – D serum	Rh type
	Positive		Negative

FIG. 7-1   Blood typing reactions.

that the full number of 168 genes will be identified in these series. The antigens are classified as HLA, human leukocyte antigens.

The importance of these antigens is related to the following conditions or diseases:

Febrile reactions to transfusion in sensitized individuals
Leukopenia (adult and neonatal)
Transplant rejection
Studies of parentage and genetics
Acute leukemias, systemic lupus erythematosus, Hodgkin's disease

Platelet

Several platelet antigens have been identified: P1-A1, P1-E1, P1-A2, Ko^a, and Ko^b. Although the current status of use of platelet-antigen studies is still in the research realm, it is expected that clinical use will be found in clarifying etiology of neonatal thrombocytopenic purpura in relation to maternal antibodies and in explaining some of the drug-induced thrombocytopenias.

COOMBS' TESTS

The Coombs' tests are valuable tools in differentiating between types of hemolytic anemias, in detecting immune antibodies that may be present in the serum of a transfusion recipient, and in testing for an anticipated erythroblastotic infant. One of these tests (direct Coombs') is done to check red blood cells for the presence of antibodies that coat the cells without completing the reaction of agglutination. The other (indirect Coombs') is done on serum to test for presence of antibodies to the red blood cell antigens.

Direct Coombs' test is used in studies of acquired hemolytic anemia and to test the umbilical cord blood of an erythroblastotic infant. In many hospitals, direct Coombs' tests are done routinely on *all* cord bloods, regardless of whether the infant appears affected or not. This picks up any sensitizations that are not obvious but might develop within a few days after delivery.

Indirect Coombs' test is used in transfusion cross matches and to detect the presence of anti-Rh antibodies in maternal serum before delivery.

BLOOD TRANSFUSIONS

General Considerations

The transfusion of blood from one person to another is a tissue transplant, which is a serious matter. It is recognized universally that there is no satisfactory substitute for whole blood when the need for it is indicated. On the other hand, unless the hazards attendant to its use are constantly kept in mind, this lifesaving substance can do more harm than good and can on occasion kill. The hazards include hemolytic transfusion reaction, homologous serum jaundice, circulatory overload, pyrogenic reaction, and allergic and anaphylactoid reaction. There must be careful attention to detail in each step of the preparation and administration of blood. The role of the nurse is vital: He must be alert to avoid possible slips on his part that could lead to serious consequences, and he must be alert during and after transfusion to detect any changes in the patient that could be attributed to the transfusion process.

Concerned because there was increasing evidence of indiscriminate use of blood transfusions, the Joint Blood Council and American Association of Blood Banks recommended basic criteria for blood transfusion in 1962. The recommendations specified the uses to be made of whole blood and blood fractions, outlining the indications for all the uses to be made of the products involved in the light of physiopathologic states and the hydrodynamics of circulation. When transfusion is considered, the first question to be answered is, "What deficiency is to be corrected?" and the correct choice can then be made. Table 7-4 on page 197 summarizes the pertinent points to be considered. The wisdom of using packed red blood cells in chronic anemia, for example, is seen when one recognizes that the deficiency is in the oxygen-carrying capacity of the blood, for total blood volume is at normal levels. Blood-component therapy is discussed in detail later in this chapter.

Procedure

Identification of the recipient and the sample of his blood used for the typing and cross match must be absolutely correct. The request for a transfusion should be filled out completely and should include information regarding previous transfusions as well as the history of pregnancies. The blood samples must be collected in stoppered tubes, with identification of patient and date on the label, which is firmly attached to the tube. In case of any doubt regarding identification of the patient or the blood sample, another specimen should be obtained.

Cross Match

The recipient's blood type and Rh factor are determined, and the appropriate blood is selected from the blood bank. Before blood may be safely administered, an accurate cross match of donor and recipient serums and cells must be carried out. The cross match establishes compatibility between the specific donor and recipient bloods. Compatibility is shown by the absence of clumping when serums and cells are appropriately mixed and incubated. The major cross match is that between recipient serum and donor cells; the minor is that between recipient cells and donor serum. Individual cross matches rule out the possibility of antibodies developed by the recipient to bloods other than his own and serve as a check on the typing procedure for donor and recipient. When more than one unit of blood is given at a time, cross matches between donor bloods are also performed.

Essential Steps Preliminary to Transfusion

When the cross match has been completed and the unit (or units) of blood is ready to be dispensed, the unit is labeled with the recipient's name and hospital number and the signature of the person who performed the cross match. A form giving complete information concerning the recipient and donor types and the cross-match tests done, as well as a report of the serologic test for syphilis done on the donor blood, is attached to the patient's chart.

Before starting the transfusion, the blood is inspected for hemolysis and abnormal cloudiness or color. When the blood is judged satisfactory, it is gently and thoroughly mixed. The only medication that is allowed to be given with blood is blood-group-specific substances (A and/or B), as indicated.

Before starting the transfusion, the person administering the blood must check for correct identification of the recipient and the unit of blood prepared for him. When the recipient is anesthetized or unconscious, great care is essential in identification.

When units of blood prepared for a given recipient are not used, they should be returned to the blood bank for reissue. Only those units in which the container closure has not been pierced and which have been kept refrigerated at a temperature of about 5°C will be accepted for reissue.

Reactions to Transfusion

HEMOLYTIC

By far the most important of possible transfusion reactions is the hemolytic reaction. This is particularly so because it is the one most subject to human error at any point in the process of transfusion and because it is very serious in its consequences. Hemolytic reactions are most commonly caused by errors in, or inadequacy of, typing and cross-matching techniques, improper identification and labeling of specimens or units of blood, or improper identification of the recipient.

Symptoms of hemolytic reaction are fever, chills, back and leg pain, dyspnea, hypotension, urticaria, and nausea. Hemoglobinemia and hemoglobinuria will be seen within the first 2 to 4 h after a hemolytic reaction due to incompatible blood. In cases of hemolytic reaction, investigation of the cause is imperative. The remainder of the unit of blood being given at the time of reaction is returned to the laboratory for tests to discover the reason for the reaction. These tests include recheck of identification, typing, and cross matching, and checks for sterility. The patient's urine should be saved and observed for hemoglobinuria, and tests for hemoglobinemia and bilirubin should be done on the blood.

FEBRILE

The most frequent cause of febrile reaction is contamination of the blood by bacteria or, sometimes, chemicals in the apparatus used to collect or administer the blood. Another possible source of febrile reaction is the antigenic activity of the donor leukocytes or platelets. For patients known to have a sensitivity to these cells, the buffy coat is removed before the transfusion is started.

Symptoms of febrile reaction are fever and/or chills and occasionally lumbar pain.

ALLERGIC

Although usually mild, allergic reaction can be serious. In patients with known hypersensitivity, Benadryl, given in conjunction with the administration of blood (but not *with the blood*), has prevented or minimized allergic reaction.

Symptoms of allergic reaction include urticaria, bronchial spasm, edema, and headache or dizziness.

CIRCULATORY OVERLOAD

When blood is administered too fast and in too large an amount, left heart failure can be a serious complication of transfusion therapy. This is particularly true in patients with chronic anemia or hypoproteinemia. Pulmonary congestion and edema result from circulatory overload.

Intravenous Fluids and Administration of Blood

When intravenous infusions of solutions are given, the various solutions used are readily diluted as they enter the circulation drop by drop. From this, it is seen that such solutions may be considered compatible with blood. Conversely, when small amounts of blood are mixed with most solutions, there is an "incompatibility" in that clotting or hemolysis due to the hypertonicity of the solution may occur. Such a situation results from the mixing of medications with blood being transfused, and this is the rationale behind the prohibition of giving medications by mixture with blood. Isotonic sodium chloride is the *only* solution which is "compatible" in the sense being used here. Intravenous solutions containing calcium (Ringer's, lactated Ringer's, and many of the balanced solutions) have the potential of causing citrated blood to clot. If there is to be a change from a calcium-containing solution to blood or vice versa, the tubing must be flushed with normal (isotonic) saline before and after the blood is given.

Hints on Administration Blood[1]

1. Flow calculations are based on the following: milliliters of fluid wanted divided by minutes of infusion wanted equals milliliters

[1] From "The Use of Blood," Abbott Laboratories, North Chicago, Ill., 1965. By permission.

per minute. The milliliters per minute multiplied by drops per milliliter (for the administration set you are using) equals the number of drops per minute to give.

2. Make sure you have only the designated blood or solution. Make sure you have the right patient. Take nothing for granted. Do not rely on color of labels or of solutions for identification. Read the labels.

3. Red cells settle to the bottom; plasma rises to the top. Whole blood should be mixed well before starting the infusion and gently agitated from time to time during transfusion for trouble-free flow.

4. When setting up a glass blood bottle for administration, insert the airway needle immediately after starting transfusion. This technique clears any blood present in the air tube. However, *never use an airway needle with a plastic container.* If the plastic drip chamber of a blood-administration set assumes an hourglass shape, the airway is plugged. Replace airvent needle.

5. Administer the first 50 ml of blood slowly for 30 min and watch the patient continuously for 15 min for any signs of reactions.

6. Check flow rates frequently. Changing height of the stand or bed during administration may alter an established rate. Other factors altering flow rate: repositioning the extremity undergoing transfusion; temporarily halting the procedure; changes in location of needle in vein; changes in tone of the vein.

SELECTION AND SCREENING OF BLOOD DONORS

Selection of Blood Donors

Blood banks must depend in large measure on the relatives and friends of recipients to replace the blood used. Even with the advantage of decreasing the cost to the recipient by replacing the blood used, it is characteristic of all blood banks that more blood is dispensed than is supplied by this means. Careful screening of blood donors is absolutely necessary to protect the donor himself as well as the recipient. The Scientific Committee of the Joint Blood

Council, Inc., and the Standards Committee of the American Association of Blood Banks have set up standards by which the selection of donors is made. These standards are listed below.

When a prospective donor desires to know what is required of him before he can qualify to donate blood, these standards should be explained to him. He may also want to know what to expect when he gives blood. He should have no reaction to the process physically, but there is a possibility that he may experience a psychologic reaction, because the drawing of a pint of his blood is an important event. The donor is given light refreshment after the blood is drawn, and he is expected to rest for a short time afterward to allow for the physiologic readjustment that may be necessary. The time required for drawing blood rarely exceeds 15 to 20 min. There is little, if any, pain involved in the process.

Screening of Blood Donors

1. *Age.* 21 through 59 years. (Regulations with regard to acceptance of minors are subject to individual blood bank rulings. In general, minors 17 to 19 years of age are accepted if they have their parents' consent, if they are married, or if they are members of the Armed Forces.)
2. *Blood pressure.* Between 100 and 200 mm Hg systolic and 50 and 100 mm Hg diastolic. (Regulations with regard to acceptance of hypertensive persons may vary with different blood banks. Some use these persons when they have the written approval of the physician who is treating them.)
3. *Medical limitations.* All donors must be in good health, with no upper respiratory infection and no allergic symptoms, Rejection is imperative if they have a medical history of malaria, hepatitis, jaundice, or venereal disease. No person with a history of tuberculosis should be accepted. The prospective donor must not be receiving any medication regularly. If he is under medical care, blood banks will require that his physician's written approval and statement of diagnosis be known before he will be considered.
4. *Temperature.* The body temperature should be no higher than 99.6°F.

5. *Pregnancy.* Pregnancy during the previous 6 months excludes a donor.

6. *Dental surgery.* Dental surgery or tooth extraction during the previous 72 h excludes a donor.

7. *Hemoglobin.* Minimal levels for acceptance as donors are 13.5 g for men and 12.5 g for women.

8. *Receipt of blood or blood derivatives.* Donors are rejected if there is a history of having received blood or blood products during the preceding 6 months.

9. *Food and drink.* All foods and liquids other than clear beverages must be withheld for a period of at least 3 h prior to donation. Alcoholic beverages must be withheld for this same period of time before donation.

10. *Tests performed on donor's blood.* In addition to careful determination of the donor's ABO blood type and Rh factor, a serologic test for syphilis is done. Since serum (homologous) hepatitis is transmitted via blood or materials contaminated with blood, a major concern is prevention of such an accident in blood transfusion. Seven million units of blood are given each year in the United States, and of these, in 1971, 150,000 recipients developed hepatitis. In 1971, the Bureau of Biologic Standards instituted the requirement that donor bloods be tested for the presence of the hepatitis B antigen (HBA_g). Although not fully capable of identifying possible hepatitis carriers, the HAA (hepatitis-associated antigen) serologic test is extremely important as a screening test to reduce the incidence of transfusion-associated hepatitis. The development of the radioimmunoassay HAA procedure offers better promise of specificity and sensitivity. One of the consequences of this problem is that most hospitals now require the patient to sign a consent form for transfusion. Another consequence is that, in Illinois, for example, a law has been enacted requiring blood to be labeled as having been donated by a volunteer or paid donor, since HAA incidence in the latter (particularly related to donor populations of unknown background) has been found to be significantly higher.

BLOOD COMPONENTS

The history of blood transfusion provides an excellent example of the gains made possible by devoted work combined with insight, knowledge, and increasingly precise instrumentation. The gains are more far-reaching than appears at first glance, for work on immunohematologic problems has applicability to many aspects of the basic sciences in medicine. As noted earlier, transfusion of blood and blood fractions are matters for judicious use, with therapy focused on the principal problem presented by the patient. Table 7-4 summarizes the indications for, and uses of, blood components.

Collection, Preservation, and Storage of Blood

Specially prepared plastic bags containing the appropriate anticoagulant, preservative, and nutrient for red cells are used to receive blood from the donor. The bags have a capacity of about 500 ml, including the solution. The routine solution is A-C-D—acid-citrate-dextrose. Citric acid is a general preservative, trisodium citrate the anticoagulant, and dextrose the nutrient for red cells. Heparin is used as the anticoagulant for special purposes, such as priming heart-lung machines. Since its anticoagulant properties are short-lived, such a unit must be used with 12 h of collection.

Blood for transfusion purposes must be stored in a refrigerator carefully set and monitored to maintain a temperature of 40°F (5°C). With the preservative solution and low temperature, blood may be stored for up to 3 weeks. With aging, there is a shift of sodium and potassium ions between solution/plasma and the intracellular environment, and the dextrose nutrient eventually is exhausted. Outdated units of blood may be used to prepare some of the fractions discussed below.

Blood Fractions
PACKED RED CELLS

Through either the natural settling-out process or centrifugation, cells are concentrated in the lower half of the unit. About two-thirds

TABLE 7-4   EXAMPLES OF USES OF BLOOD COMPONENTS

Blood components	Uses
Whole blood	Hypovolemic shock Acute blood loss
Leukocyte-poor units	Multiple transfusions Organ transplants
Frozen red cells	Autotransfusion Rare-blood-types inventory Rare antigens for identification of antibodies Leukocyte-poor units
Albumin	Shock Severe protein loss Hyperbilirubinemia Toxic conditions
Packed red cells	Chronic anemia Exchange transfusion in hemolytic disease of the newborn Priming renal dialysis and extracorporeal heart-lung units
Platelets	Thrombocytopenia
Cryoprecipitate	Hemophilia
γ-Globulin	Agammaglobulinemia Hypogammaglobulinemia
Immune serum γ-globulins	Specific for disease prophylaxis or modification

of the plasma is drawn off, so that the hematocrit of the remaining suspension is 60 to 70 percent. Since this range of hematocrit tends to produce greater viscosity, there will be slower flow in transfusion. Sterile balanced salt solution may be added to resuspend the cells in a concentration of 40 to 50 percent. This is particularly preferred when the use is to be priming renal dialysis or heart-lung machines.

Packed red cells minimize risk of circulatory overload or cardio-vascular failure. In addition, better balance of sodium, potassium, and ammonium ions is maintained, and citrate overdose prevented. With removal of plasma, the antibody content is reduced markedly, an advantage in transfusion of sensitized patients and a preventive measure in patients needing frequent transfusions.

Human serum albumin may be added to the packed cells prepared for exchange transfusion in treating hemolytic disease of the newborn. This provides a source of protein to which excess bilirubin can be bound, thus alleviating the strain on the infant's system.

LEUKOCYTE-POOR UNITS

There are approximately 3 to 4 billion leukocytes in a unit of blood. It is impossible to reduce this population to much less than 2 million, the range usually being up to 3 million. The highest incidence and levels of leukocyte antibodies occur in patients who receive frequent transfusions, multiparous women, and tissue transplants. The reaction with incompatible leukocytes is not life-threatening, as is that of incompatible red cells. It resembles the pyrogenic reaction. Within about 5 min of exposure, the patient may experience flushing, palpitation, tightness in the chest, cough, and a slight rise in temperature. Subsequent manifestations include increased diastolic pressure, headache, malaise, elevated temperature, sometimes accompanied by chills. The blood differential count shows a neutrophilic shift to the left.

Several methods of preparing leukocyte-poor units of blood are in use: centrifugation, nylon filtration, dextran sedimentation, saline washing, and reconstituting frozen red cells. With removal of the buffy coat after centrifugation, red cells are also drawn off. Nylon filtration is not advisable for use in tissue transplants because lymphocytes tend to be retained. Dextran sedimentation causes clumping of the leukocytes, and the unit must be used within 3 h. (This method does not yet have Federal Drug Administration approval for general use.) Saline washing is cumbersome, relatively inefficient in removing leukocytes, and demands the utmost in sterile techniques.

Reconstitution of frozen red cells obviously assumes their availability, which is rather limited at present.

FROZEN RED CELLS

The first step in preparation of blood for freezing is conglomeration of the red cells in loose, but fairly large, aggregates by the gradual addition of glycerol and mechanical concentration. The glycerol protects the red cells from rupture when frozen. The prepared unit is rapidly frozen, at -80°C or below, and maintained at this temperature. When it is to be used, the cell pack is thawed, the glycerol is removed by serial washing, and the unit is then reconstituted to the desired concentration with balanced salt solution. The special technique and equipment required for preparing and freezing blood imposes limitations on its availability. Frozen red cells may be stored for long periods.

The uses of frozen red cells are listed in Table 7-4. This method makes it possible to maintain inventories of selected types of red cells which are less common. Since there is no plasma involved, there is no introduction of antibodies on transfusion. For individuals who have very rare types or unidentified antibodies that make it difficult to find compatible donors, blood may be drawn and frozen in anticipation of later need associated with elective surgery, etc. for autotransfusion.

PLATELETS

Individuals who have either quantitative lack of platelets (thrombocytopenia) or whose platelets are qualitatively deficient (thromboasthenia) may require transfusion to supply sufficient numbers of these important participants in the coagulation process. When whole blood is used, the number of units which may be given is limited because of strain on volume capacity. Transfusions of platelet-rich plasma or platelet concentrates is the treatment of choice when bleeding occurs in response to a platelet count less than $10,000/mm^3$. There should be an increase of 12,000 to 15,000 in the count following this treatment. Platelet-rich preparations are half the volume of whole blood and retain 90 percent of the platelets in fresh blood. Platelet concentrates provide 70 to 80 percent of the platelets in fresh blood in a volume of 25 ml. Because of their property of cohesiveness, platelets must be administered with non-wettable infusion sets which include an 80-μm mesh nonwettable filter and nonwettable needle. The blood bank should be notified in advance of the need for these types of blood components because of the special preparation required and because they must be used in less than 6 h after drawing.

CRYOPRECIPITATE

The most common bleeding problem is that due to deficiency in factor VIII (antihemophilic globulin). J. G. Pool and A. E. Shannon developed a method of isolating factor VIII from plasma by a precipitation process involving freezing (indicated by the name for this blood component). Quantitation of the effectiveness of this concentrate is based on a unit defined as the amount necessary to raise the activity of one deciliter of deficient plasma one percent or as the activity present in one milliliter normal fresh plasma. Dosage is calculated on the basis of the patient's weight or plasma volume. Cryoprecipitate is packaged in 3-ml amounts with a notation of the unit content.

Example of Calculation of Dose

A patient with 2,600 ml plasma volume has less than 1-percent factor-VIII activity. In order to raise the activity to 30 percent, the following equation is used to calculate the dose needed:

Activity desired x plasma volume = units required
0.20 x 2,600 = 780 units

The number of units required is divided by the number of units per bag:

780/130 = 6 = no. of bags required

TABLE 7-5   COMPOSITION OF CRYOPRECIPITATE

Factor	Name	Amount, %
VIII	Antihemophilic globulin	56
I	Fibrinogen	23
II	Prothrombin	1.5
V	Proaccelerin	1.0
VII	Proconvertin	1.8
IX	Plasma thromboplastin component	5.5
X	Stuart-Prower	1.4
XI	Plasma thromboplastin antecedent	1.1
XII	Hageman	2.0

SOURCE: From "Blood Component Therapy," American Association of Blood Banks, Chicago, 1969.

Cryoprecipitate must be used within 3 h of thawing. The usual priming dose is twice the amount calculated, with maintenance doses given every 12 h thereafter until the bleeding is brought under control.

PLASMA PROTEINS

Albumin is prepared in concentrations of 5% in buffered saline, and 25% in salt-poor diluent. It may be used in treatment of shock due to hemorrhage, trauma, or infection. If plasma is not available on demand, albumin may be used as replacement of lost plasma proteins, which is associated with severe burns. In hypoproteinemia, it may be given for supportive or symptomatic treatment.

Fibrinogen is supplied as a dry powder which must be reconstituted very carefully to avoid foaming and denaturation. The usual amount per vial is 1 to 2 g; the vial often carries the label "clottable protein." Dosage is calculated on clottable-protein content and clinical assessment of need. The use of fibrinogen carries a high risk of transmission of hepatitis (as much as 25 percent); it is therefore to be used with great caution. It is recommended that a prophylactic dose of 10 ml γ-globulin be given within the week following the use of fibrinogen and once again 4 weeks after the first dose. Not only must the patient be protected, but those who handle fibrinogen products must avoid exposure via needle scratches, small cuts, etc. If exposure does occur, a prophylactic dose of γ-globulin is required.

γ-Globulin (nonspecific) is used in treatment of agammaglobulinemia and hypogammaglobulinemia. When specific antibodies are present, the amount may be designated according to the particular disease. These diseases include measles, poliomyelitis, infectious hepatitis, tetanus, pertussis, mumps, or vaccinia. (Treatment of Rh sensitization, which also uses γ-globulin, is discussed later in this chapter.) Table 7-6 summarizes the dosages required.

Dextran is a polysaccharide of glucose units with a molecular weight of 70,000. It is a synthetic plasma substitute which functions in the maintenance of oncotic pressure. Its primary uses are as an emergency treatment for acute hemorrhage or burn shock until more definitive blood components can be given. It offers the advantages of being inexpensive, readily available, and of carrying no risk of transmitting hepatitis. It may interfere with cross-match tests and may cause coagulation defects. Allergic reactions have also been reported.

PLASMAPHERESIS

Plasmapheresis is a procedure in which blood is drawn, the plasma separated from the cells, and the cells returned to the individual. It requires special closed-system equipment in order to maintain strict sterility throughout all the steps in the process. The blood is drawn into a bag that contains anticoagulant and to which is attached a satellite bag for collection of plasma. Other satellite bags may be used for particular blood fractions in addition to plasma.

Indications for plasmapheresis in treatment of disease are (*a*) circulatory overload, (*b*) macroglobulinemia, and (*c*) plasma exchange to rid the blood of toxic substances associated with hepatic coma, drugs, or chemicals. In circulatory overload, the problem is hypervolemia. By plasmapheresis, the blood volume is reduced, but cell content is maintained. Plasma exchange is used in reducing the

TABLE 7-6   DOSAGES OF γ-GLOBULIN

Disease	Amount	Time
Agammaglobulinemia Hypoglobulinemia	0.2–0.5 ml/lb body wt	2–4 week intervals
Poliomyelitis	0.14 ml/lb body wt	As soon as possible if history of immunization is doubtful or absent
Measles	0.1 ml/lb body wt (prophylaxis) 0.02 ml/lb body wt (modification)	Within 6 days of exposure
Infectious hepatitis	0.01–0.02 ml/lb body wt	Passive protection subsides in a few weeks
Tetanus	Adults: 250 units Children: 2 units/lb body wt	As soon as possible
Pertussis	1.5 ml	As soon as possible after exposure, followed by 2 doses per week. With symptoms, every 1 to 2 days until convalescence
Mumps	90 lb body wt: 1.5 ml 90–140 lb: 3.0 ml More than 140 lb; 4.5 ml	Within 1 week of exposure; for treatment to modify disease, larger amounts determined by clinical course
Vaccinia	0.15 ml/lb body wt (prophylaxis) 0.3 ml/lb body wt (in serious complications)	As soon as possible

SOURCE: From "Blood Component Therapy," American Association of Blood Banks, 1969.

concentration of macroglobulins and in flushing exogenous and endogenous toxic material from the blood.

With increasing sophistication in the use of blood components, plasmapheresis provides the means to obtain these important elements that only the human body can produce. The body can tolerate the loss of protein and fluids in the unit proportion used (approximately 5 dl) at more frequent intervals because these elements are readily replenished naturally. Blood cells are not readily replenished. Plasma donations at weekly intervals up to four times are permissible if the donor's serum protein is maintained above 6 g/dl.

HEMOLYTIC DISEASE OF THE NEWBORN

Etiology and Characteristics

Hemolytic disease of the newborn (HDN), also called erythroblastosis fetalis, is a disease characterized by intravascular hemolysis of the infant's cells during gestation, caused by antibodies from the maternal system. Two possibilities for sensitization of the mother exist. She may have received transfusion of incompatible [e.g., Rh_0 (D)-positive] blood as the initiating event.[1] If this initial sensitization occurred before any pregnancy, all subsequent pregnancies would have an equal chance of resulting in an affected infant if the father had a blood factor incompatible with the mother. The other mechanism of sensitization is by a "fetal bleed" into the maternal circulation. This may occur during gestation as a result of a placental leak, allowing fetal cells to enter the maternal circulation. The most frequent fetal bleeds are thought to be at delivery when the placenta separates from the uterine wall. This helps to explain the common observation that a normal infant may be delivered of a primipara, but subsequent pregnancies result in HDN. How the mother's Rh antibodies reach the fetus is not understood. For despite the fact that antibodies are molecules much smaller than red blood cells—small enough infact, to cross the placenta—some means of cellular

[1] Gorman cites a rare example of what he termed "initiation by initiation" in which a "ceremony" of mixing small amounts of blood of sorority pledges resulted in the sensitization of one member.

transport is required for antibodies of the immune type to enter the fetal circulation.

When there is excessive destruction of red cells, the fetal system responds with the release of immature cells (erythroblasts) which are seen in the smears of newborn peripheral blood. This finding gave the name erythroblastosis fetalis to the disease. Prior to the development of hematologic examinations, the disease was recognized and named neonatal icterus gravis. Both of these terms are descriptive only. When the anemia is severe, there is proliferation of extra-medullary blood-forming tissue, and this, along with the demands made upon the liver and spleen, accounts for hepatosplenomegaly common to the disease in severe form.

Statistically, it has been found that HDN resulting from incompatible matings occurs at the rate of about 0.5 percent of all deliveries of an obstetrical service. In 55 percent of these matings, the Rh-positive man will be heterozygous, and up to half (and possibly more) of the offspring can be Rh_0 (D)-negative. These factors of probability reduce the chances of this type of HDN. There is also a protective feature in the major blood groups of the parents. If the major blood groups are incompatible (e.g., father, group A; mother, group B) and the fetus inherits the father's group, cells from the fetal bleed will be destroyed by the naturally occurring agglutinins of the mother. This reduces the probability of initiation of antibody response to near zero.

In addition to sensitization with an Rh factor or one of the

TABLE 7-7   LABORATORY AIDS TO DIAGNOSIS AND
MANAGEMENT OF HEMOLYTIC DISEASE OF THE
NEWBORN

Blood group genotyping
Antibody titers
Direct Coombs' test
Bilirubin
Amniotic-fluid analysis
Identification of fetal-cell population in maternal circulation
Newborn hemoglobin, hematocrit, differential, reticulocyte counts
Hemoglobin-type (adult and fetal) ratio

---

other types, there is, for example, the possibility of HDN when the mother is group O and the fetus is A, B, or AB. The maternal system may be stimulated to produce more agglutinin for the blood group of the fetus. HDN due to ABO incompatibility is milder than that of other varieties.

It is now routine to check all pregnant women for their blood group and Rh genotype as part of the initial examination in pre-natal care. If the patient is Rh-negative, her serum is checked for antibodies. If antibodies are found, the husband's blood group and Rh genotype are determined to provide clues for the identification of the antibodies. By the beginning of the third trimester, a second antibody titer is done to detect a possible rise in titer.

Amniotic-fluid Analysis

In addition to the antibody titers, modern management of known immunization has developed greater precision by the use of analyses of amniotic fluid. When the antibody titer exceeds 1:32, amniotic-fluid analysis is indicated as a means of assessing the status of the fetus. If there is a hemolytic process going on, the amniotic fluid will be altered, as determined by chemical and/or spectrophotometric analysis. Especially in serial determinations, the degree of change determines the necessity for intrauterine transfusion or, if gestation has progressed far enough, the necessity for induction of labor. For detailed discussion of the techniques and nursing roles, the references given at the end of the chapter are highly recommended. Table 7-8 summarizes the relationship between amniotic-fluid analysis and indications for transfusion or induction of labor.

Intrauterine Transfusion

When intrauterine transfusion is needed, blood compatible with the mother (usually group O, Rh_0 (D)-negative) is used from packed-cell preparation. Preparing the patient for the procedure involves the radiology department, since the target area in the fetus is the abdominal cavity. (Cells are absorbed into the fetal circulation from this site via the lymphatic channels into the great veins.) The fetal abdominal cavity is located by fluoroscopy. A liquid radiopaque contrast me-

TABLE 7-8   INTERPRETATION OF AMNIOTIC-FLUID ANALYSIS

Change in OD reading	Freda Classification	Equivalent bilirubin mg/dl level	Clinical significance	Indicated management
<0.20	1+ (abnormal)	<0.25	Normal, mildly affected, or Rh neg. baby	Plan to deliver at 38 weeks
0.20–0.34	2+ (abnormal)	0.28–0.46	Rh-pos. baby; affected but not in immediate danger	Repeat exam in 7 days
0.34–0.70	3+	0.46–0.94	Rh-pos. baby; distressed probably in failure	Intrauterine transfusion if before 32 weeks; immediate delivery if 33 weeks or more
>0.70	4+ (abnormal)	>0.95	Rh-pos. baby; impending fetal death	Immediate delivery

SOURCE: Adapted from J. G. Gorman, "The Role of the Laboratory in Hemolytic Disease of the Newborn," Lea & Febiger, Philadelphia. In press.

dium is injected into the amniotic cavity and after 24 h (during which time the fetus will have swallowed the contrast medium, the fetal abdomen is located in relation to radiopaque tape markers placed on the mother's abdomen, using the fluoroscope. Under local anesthetic, a 17-gauge thin-walled Tuohy needle is inserted, and entrance into the fetal abdominal cavity is made. A catheter is inserted through the needle, and the needle is removed. Further assurance of the site is made by injecting a small amount of contrast medium through the catheter to coat the peritoneal surface. The transfusion is then completed.

Prevention of Sensitization

With the combination of fuller understanding of the immunologic mechanisms of HDN and availability of specific immune γ-globulin, the means to prevent development of maternal antibodies to Rh_0 D^u antigens has been realized. The key is Rh_0GAM,[1] the immune human globulin. The goal of complete elimination of Rh hemolytic disease has been defined in the following quotation from the introduction to a symposium held in New York in 1969.[2]

> It is estimated that there are 300,000 sensitized Rh-negative mothers in the childbearing age in the United States. These mothers contribute all of the cases of Rh hemolytic disease in this country. If no new mothers enter this pool, the number of sensitized Rh negative mothers in the United States would gradually dwindle and Rh hemolytic disease would virtually disappear in one generation. Rh_0GAM Rh_0 (D) Immune Globulin (Human), used whenever an Rh negative woman is in danger of becoming sensitized to the Rh_0 (D) antigen, would prevent any new sensitizations from occurring, and thereby relegate Rh hemolytic disease to a disease of the past.

Rh_0GAM provides for suppression of the development of antibody if it is administered within 72 h after delivery. The rationale is based on the immunologic principle of passive immunization. The anti-Rh_0 globulin "clears" the maternal system of fetal blood cells carrying the Rh factor before the maternal system is sensitized, i.e., responds to the foreign antigen by synthesizing antibodies. Use of Rh_0GAM is guided by the criteria listed in the product description, all of which must be met. They describe the status of the mother and baby as follows:

1. She is Rh_0 (D)- and D^u-negative.
2. She has not been immunized to the Rh_0 (D) factor.
3. She has delivered a baby who is either Rh_0 (D)-positive for D^u-positive.

Unless the father is known to be Rh_0 (D)-negative and D^u-negative, the fetus of a miscarriage should be assumed to have been positive, and treatment with Rh_0GAM should be instituted if the other two criteria are met.

---

[1] Rh_0GAM is the product of Ortho Diagnostics, Raritan, N.J.
[2] Rh_0GAM One Year Later," p. 3, Ortho Diagnostics, Raritan, N.J., 1969.

PRELIMINARY TESTS

Several tests are required in preparation for the administration of Rh_0 GAM. These include:

1. Confirmation of maternal Rh_0 (D) and D^u status
2. Cross-match of maternal cells with Rh_0 GAM
3. Direct Coombs' test on mother's and baby's cells
4. Estimate of fetal-cell population in the mother's blood

The first test is necessary to meet the first criterion of indications for use of Rh_0 GAM. If a positive results, its use is ruled out. In the second test, a 1:1,000 dilution of the specific lot of Rh_0GAM is used. This dilution is supplied with each package of the drug. There should be no clumping of the cells. If there is, it may be due to the cells' having been coated with antibody (positive direct Coombs' test), D^u-positive cells, or a large fetal-cell population. The first two possibilities demonstrate a check on the other tests. In the third, it is reasonable to expect that fetal cells, being positive, would react with the immune globulin. This would not rule out giving Rh_0 GAM, but it is essential to confirm the level of fetal-cell population by other means before proceeding with treatment. If the direct Coombs' test is positive for either the mother's or baby's cells, this is confirmatory evidence of the presence of antibody in the maternal system and rules out giving Rh_0GAM. Estimation of fetal-cell population in the mother's blood is useful in explaining an incompatible Rh_0 GAM cross-match if the other tests are in line, and it may also be used in determining the need for additional treatment. Following administration of the drug, a test to determine the passively acquired antibody titer is performed at specified intervals up to 3 months postpartum.

TREATMENT

The usual dose of Rh_0GAM is 300 μg (1 vial). The laboratory dispenses the drug. As noted above, it must be given within 72 h after delivery. It is given to the postpartum patient only; it must *not* be given to the infant. The injection must be intramuscular. Contraindications include (*a*) an Rh_0 (D)- or D^u-positive mother, (*b*) one who has received Rh_0 (D)-positive blood transfusion within 3 months, and (c) one who has been previously immunized to Rh_0 (D). Reactions to the drug are infrequent and generally mild.

It should be noted that, simple as the procedure appears to be, there remain questions to be answered, and individual differences in patients that pose problems. These will be resolved with the help of thorough records, even more precise tests, and sound clinical judgment. The latter is particularly important in evaluating individiual patient needs for increasing the dosage.

Since the drug is expensive, the decision to use it is usually left up to the patient after her physician explains the implications of Rh_0 (D) sensitization and the goals of treatment. Although the primary concern focuses on protection of subsequent pregnancies, another important consideration relates to protection against transfusion problems, should the patient need this treatment any time later in life and inadvertantly be transfused with Rh-positive blood. While such a mistake is increasingly being avoided, it still could happen with life-threatening results. It is common practice to require patients who refuse treatment to sign a release in order to protect the physician and laboratory from malpractice suit if she later encounters problems stemming from Rh immunization.

EXCHANGE TRANSFUSION

Exchange transfusion is, as noted in the section on packed red cells, used in a number of cases. The discussion which follows is focused on its use in treating neonatal hyperbilirubinemia, since this is by far the most common use. The primary objective is to rid the infant's system of the excessive bilirubin burden and thus prevent kernicterus. Exchange transfusions involve the simultaneous administration of blood free from the antigen that causes the disease and removal of blood of the infant. It is, in effect, a flushing procedure. The infant's own blood-cell-producing tissues will continue to release cells of his established type, of course. Since the life span of red blood cells is about 120 days, his blood will be completely of his own manufacture after that time, despite the exchange transfusion. Since bilirubin bound to serum albumin does not cross the blood-brain barrier, it may be used in the suspension of packed red cells to give the infant this additional protection.

REFERENCES

"Blood Component Therapy," American Association of Blood Banks, Chicago, 1969.

Brittingham, T. E., and H. Chaplin, Jr.: Febrile Transfusion Reactions Caused by Sensitivity to Donor Leukocytes and Platelets, *JAMA*, **165**:823, 1957.

Dausset, J., L. Colombain, N. Legrand, N. Feingold, and F. T. Rappaport: Genetic and Biological Aspects of HL-A System of Human Histocompatibility, *Blood*, **35**:591, 1970.

Davidsohn, Israel, and John B. Henry (eds.): "Todd-Sanford Clinical Diagnosis by Laboratory Methods," 15th ed., Saunders, Philadelphia, 1974.

Freda, Vincent J., and J. G. Robertson: Amniotic Fluid Analysis in Rh Isoimmunization, *Amer. J. Nurs.*, **65**(8):64, 1965.

Glynn, Elizabeth: Nursing Support during Intra-uterine Transfusion, *Amer. J. Nurs.*, **65**(8):72, 1965.

Huestis, D. S., J. R. Bove, and S. Busch: "Practical Blood Transfusion," Little, Brown, Boston, 1969.

Levine, Phillip: The Influence of the ABO System on Rh Hemolytic Disease, *Hum. Biol.*, **30**(2):14, 1958.

Milic, Ann, and Kalis Adamsons: Fetal Blood Sampling, *Amer. J. Nurs.*, **68**:2149–2152, 1968.

Pool, J. G., and A. E. Shannon: Production of High-potency Concentrates of Anti-hemophilic Globulin in a Closed-bag System, *New Eng. J. Med.*, **273**:1443–1447, 1965.

Queenan, John T.: "Modern Management of Rh Problems," Harper & Row, New York, 1967.

"Standards for a Blood Transfusion Service," 5th ed., American Association of Blood Banks, Chicago, 1971/72.

Sussman, L. N.: "Blood Grouping Tests. Medicolegal Uses," Charles C Thomas, Springfield, Ill., 1968.

"Technical Methods and Procedures," 5th ed., American Association of Blood Banks, Chicago, 1970.

Terasaki, P.I.: "Histocompatibility Testing 1970," Williams & Wilkins, Baltimore, 1970.

Woodrow, J.C.: Rh Immunization and Its Prevention, *Ser. Haematol.*, **3**:3, 1970.

EIGHT

MICROBIOLOGIC EXAMINATIONS

An understanding of microbiology is important in planning the care of patients with infectious diseases, in protecting oneself and others from infection, and in facilitating diagnosis by proper collection of the appropriate specimens. In addition, knowledge of the fundamental processes by which identification of organisms is made provides better understanding of what to expect from the laboratory and how to make use of the information derived from microbiologic studies. For example, in almost all cases, the report of a direct smear gives tentative information to be confirmed on the basis of culture studies. The time required for definitive identification of organisms is at least 24 h and often more when subcultures on special media must be made from a pure culture or from a colony of a single organism. Similarly, tests for sensitivity of the organism to antibiotic or chemotherapeutic agents must be made from pure cultures.

The material presented in this chapter is not intended to be an all-inclusive review of microbiology; rather, it is selected information which seems most pertinent to cooperation with the laboratory and to a basic understanding of infectious diseases and means of control.

PRINCIPLES OF STERILIZATION

Physical Agents

In all instances, no matter what the means being used, the *intensity* or concentration of the agent and the *time* of exposure are the important factors in sterilization. For example, heat used must be hot enough and applied long enough to bring about death of the organisms. In almost all cases, the cellular component which is altered by treatment, and thus brings about the death of the cell, is protein. When protein alteration is not accomplished, rupture of the cell is the desired effect; it can be produced by certain physical agents.

TEMPERATURE

Low temperature usually produces dormancy in the organisms rather than killing them. Exceptions to this rule are the gonococcus and meningococcus, which are sensitive to low temperatures. Freezing alone may kill many organisms, but not all of them. Alternate freeze-thaw results in cell rupture. If the organisms are subjected to drying as well as freezing, (lyophilizing) cells are preserved.

Heat is one of the most common means of sterilization and is applied in both moist and dry conditions. The time required for each of these conditions is different, however. Moist heat requires a temperature of 120°C for 15 min to kill organisms, including the more resistant spores. Dry heat, on the other hand, requires 160°C for 60 min. Moist heat is more effective than dry heat, since, with a high water content of the atmosphere, penetration of steam is enhanced, and the heat of condensation of steam provides better conduction of heat than does air. Heat alters protein structure, eventually resulting in coagulation of the protein. Water is involved in this, since it has been shown that the polar groups of protein are immobilized with reduced water content in the protein medium. For example, a temperature of 75 to 80°C will coagulate egg albumin, but when the water content is reduced to 6 percent of the natural amount, a temperature of 145°C is required for the coagulation of this protein. Dry heat produces plasmolytic effects, which are caused by an increase in the concentration of salts in the cell, as well as oxidative effects.

DESICCATION

Simple drying kills many organisms.

RADIATION

Ultraviolet radiation is the most damaging of the common forms of radiation. Ultraviolet radiation ruptures chemical bonds and causes new linkages to form or effects collision of other molecules through activation of the molecules.

Ionizing radiation, such as x-ray, damages cells through the absorption of energy by atoms rather than molecules. Molecules containing these atoms are then affected and become unstable. Instability of the molecules subjected to ionizing radiation may be direct, in which case the molecules of the organism are affected, or indirect, in which case the molecules of the liquid medium in which the organisms are suspended are affected. The result of this molecular activation is particularly illustrated in the effect of ionizing radiation on water. Hydrogen and hydroxyl ions are formed. Hydrogen ions are oxidizing agents and hydroxyl ions are reducing agents, both of which proceed to alter protein structure.

SONIC AND SUPERSONIC WAVES

Between 70 and 90 percent of bacteria can be destroyed by sonic waves at approximately 9,000 Hz for 1 h. The detrimental effect is a product of the formation and rupture of gas bubbles in the bacterial cells. Supersonic waves of a magnitude over 100,000 Hz destroy bacteria within 10 to 15 min. In liquid media, hydrogen peroxide is formed by sonic waves, and thus a toxic chemical is present to act upon the organisms.

PRESSURE

Bacteria can resist pressure itself, but if the pressure is suddenly released, rupture of cells occurs.

Chemical Agents

HYDROGEN AND HYDROXYL IONS

Most bacterial pathogens grow best in the neutral zone, in which there is a relative balance of hydrogen and hydroxyl ions. An excess of hydrogen ions interferes with the permeability of the cell membrane and also affects the nutrients essential for bacterial growth. Hydrogen ions can compete with inorganic nutrients such as sodium, potassium, and calcium ions. Hydroxyl ions react with surface constituents of the cell through oxidation, killing the cell. The pH of intracellular contents is altered by the passage of organic acids into the cell without dissociation, altering the optimum pH for enzyme activity.

HEAVY METALS

Mercury reacts with cellular constituents, particularly with sulfhydryl groups of proteins, rendering them inert. Similarly, silver ions react with protein and are bactericidal by reaction with sulfhydryl groups. Silver ions have a high affinity for protein.

HALOGENS

Both chlorine and iodine react with enzymes, "poisoning" them so that they are no longer functional.

PHENOLIC COMPOUNDS

High concentrations of phenolic compounds break down the cell wall, whereas lower concentrations inhibit bacterial enzymes. For example, 1% phenol allows amino acids to leak from the cell. Phenol in a concentration of 0.15% inhibits the oxidative enzymes of the cell.

FORMALDEHYDE

Formaldehyde reacts with the functional groups of proteins, replacing hydrogen or amino groups and forming methylene bridges in the molecule, resulting in denaturation.

DETERGENTS

There are wetting agents which have hydrophilic or hydrophobic functions. They concentrate on bacterial cell walls. Cationic detergents (e.g., those containing ammonia) result in the bacteria losing their negative charge and, by absorbing the positive charge of the detergent, becoming permeable to amino compounds; this causes rupture of the cell wall as osmotic pressure is altered. The cationic detergents are most active in alkaline pH and in high dilutions. Both gram-positive and gram-negative organisms are affected. Anionic detergents are most active against gram-positive organisms.

GASES

Ethylene oxide and β-propiolactone kill both spores and vegetative cells by alkylation reactions with functional groups of proteins, forming hydroxymethyl groups, resulting in denaturation.

Chemotherapeutic and Antibiotic Agents

CHEMOTHERAPEUTIC AGENTS

The general principle of the effectiveness of chemotherapeutic agents against bacteria is that of inhibition of the cell's ability to synthesize its components or essential products. For example, folic acid inhibition results in a lack of essential respiratory compounds. In a somewhat similar fashion, chemotherapeutic agents which are similar in chemical structure to natural nutrients are used by the cell in the synthesis of some of its essential proteins, resulting in inert forms. For example, the sulfa drugs compete with p-aminobenzoic acid. It was through the work done to determine the action of the sulfa drugs that the theory of competitive inhibition by metabolic analogs was proven.

ANTIBIOTIC AGENTS

Antibiotic agents differ from chemotherapeutic agents in that they are derived from naturally occurring nonpathogenic organisms. They act in one of the following ways: (1) inhibit cell-wall synthesis, (2) disrupt cell-wall permeability, or (3) inhibit protein synthesis. Antibiotics produce a secondary metabolite or introduce shunts in metabolism of the cell. Antibiotic compounds may be taken into the spores of sporulating organisms.

Antibiotics which inhibit protein synthesis include chloramphenicol, tetracycline, streptomycin, erythromycin, kanamycin, and neomycin. Those which inhibit cell-wall synthesis are oxamycin, penicillin, bacitracin, novobiocin, vancomycin, and ristocetin. Permeability of the cell membrane is affected by polymyxin, gramicidin, and tyrocidin.

Chloromycetin was isolated from a mold. It is a derivative of trichloroacetic acid. Its action is broad-spectrum and includes some some viral and rickettsial organisms. It does not prevent the uptake of metabolites and has no effect on the cell wall, but ribonucleic acid and ribosomes of the bacterial cells are abnormal because of inhibition of later steps in the synthesis of proteins.

Streptomycin kills organisms chiefly by flooding the cell with nonfunctioning protein. Its molecule binds strongly with nucleic acids and alters the specificity of amino acid incorporation into polypeptides, resulting in abnormal structures. This occurs in the ribosomes of susceptible cells. Kanamycin and neomycin also have this effect.

The effect of antibiotics on cell walls was first observed in studies of *Escherichia coli*, when it was noted that the organisms assumed a spherical, rather than rodlike, form in the presence of hypertonic saline and penicillin. When the penicillin was removed, the original rodlike form was again present.

Those antibiotics which disrupt cell-membrane permeability by denaturation of the proteins within the membrane allow leakage into and out of the cell.

RESISTANCE TO ANTIBIOTICS

The development of "drug-fastness," or resistance to antibiotic and chemotherapeutic agents, is intimately connected with genetic forces, by which mutant organisms arise which are unaffected by the action of antibiotics. Either they have systems which do not require the compounds which are analogs, or their makeup is such that they are not attacked by the denaturation processes. In addition, some organisms may escape the action of the antibiotic simply by having less permeability to the drug. There may be, as in the case of penicillin, increased destruction of the drug by enzyme action of penicillinase produced by the organism. The development of an alternate metabolic pathway which excludes drug competition is another important mutational result. With the subsidence of susceptible organisms, the resistant organisms gain ascendency and become a major problem.

Mutants may be prevented from developing by the administration of a high initial concentration of the drug in order to destroy first-stage (simplest) mutants. It is common practice to administer a combination of two independently acting drugs, so that if mutants to one of the drugs appear, they will be destroyed by the second. It is important to restrict the use of antibiotics (especially the use of the more effective drugs) to serious cases. An indiscriminant use of antibiotics can lead to the clearing of all bacterial forms, producing an environment favorable for the development of infections from fungi. In addition, without adequate challenge from the invading organism, the body does not have the opportunity to develop sufficiently high levels of natural antibodies—an important factor in any subsequent infections to which the individual may succumb.

VIRUSES

General Considerations

These submicroscopic organisms have been the subject of intensive research to discover their composition, modes of infection, and the diseases they cause. In addition, they have been valuable in the study of genetics and the nucleic acids, ribonucleic acid (RNA) and deoxyribonucleic acid (DNA).

In contrast to bacterial organisms, which are identified by morphology, staining characteristics, and biochemical differences, viruses are identified by their size, their nucleic acid, the types of lesions they produce, and their serologic characteristics. Viruses are composed of an outer protein shell, or capsid, which surrounds and protects the nucleic acid, RNA or DNA. Some viruses also have an envelope made up of lipopolysaccharide-protein complexes; this envelope is exterior to the protein shell. When the virus particle (the infective form is called a virion) enters the host cell, the capsid is attacked by cellular enzymes, and the nucleic acid is freed. The viral nucleic acid then takes over the cell's machinery and replicates itself. This sequence of events occurs when a specific disease is produced. There have been found a number of reactions between virus and host cell which do not always result in immediately observable symptoms. These are as follows:

1. With slow replication, no clinical disease develops.
2. The virus may remain latent until changes in biochemical processes within the parasitized cell develop, at which time virulence and disease develop.
3. The virus may become incorporated into the genetic structure of the cell, changing the cell's normal characteristics to those of neoplastic cells.

Host and tissue specificity are outstanding characteristics of viruses. Host specificity is clearly demonstrated in the bacteriophages, viruses which are able to infect only a certain strain of a certain genus of bacterium. Cell susceptibility to infection may depend on the chemical constitution or the configuration of some of its surface components; e.g., the invasion of myxoviruses into cells is dependent upon mucopolysaccharide receptors on the cell surface.

Nomenclature

The International Subcommittee on Virus Nomenclature determines the acceptability of proposed names for viruses as they are newly isolated. When names are not given, numbers are used for individual members within a major group (e.g., reovirus). Table 8-1 lists the classification of viruses by their nucleic acid and major groups.

The derivation of the names for the groups is of interest. The picorna group is so named because its members are small (pico) and their nucleic acid is RNA. Reovirus includes both *r*espiratory and *e*nteric *o*rganisms. Arboviruses are those which are arthropod-borne. Papovavirus derives its name from a combination of the first two letters of papilloma, polyoma, and vacuolating—all terms describ-

TABLE 8-1   CLASSIFICATION OF VIRUSES

Nucleic acid	Virus group	Size, nm	Types pathogenic to man
RNA	Picorna	17–39	Poliovirus, Coxsackie viruses A and B, echovirus, rhinovirus (common cold)
	Reovirus	74	Types 1, 2, 3
	Arbovirus	20–100	Encephalitis (many varieties)
	Myxovirus	80–200	Influenza, mumps, parainfluenza, measles, respiratory syncytial
DNA	Papovavirus	40–55	Papilloma (wart)
	Adenovirus	65–85	Common cold (28 types)
	Herpesvirus	120–180	Herpes simplex, herpes zoster, cytomegalovirus
	Poxvirus	150–300	Variola (smallpox) Varicella (chickenpox)

ing group members, all of which are oncogenic. The adenovirus group is so named because the first members of the category were isolated from adenoid and tonsillar tissue. Herpesvirus includes those viruses causing herpetic, or vesicular, lesions. The poxviruses all cause diseases with extensive skin lesions termed pox. Myxoviruses are characterized by their invasion of respiratory mucous-membrane tissues. The term echovirus is based on the first letters of the description "enteric cytopathogenic human orphan." Since this group of viruses is now known to produce many diseases, the term "orphan" could be removed; this term was primarily used because, at the time of the isolation of the virus, the diseases caused by the latter were not known.

Routes of Infection and Disease Manifestation

POXVIRUS

Among the poxviruses, the following diagram shows the pathways of infection, points of virus replication, and overt disease.

Respiratory tract

regional lymph nodes, where multiplication occurs
↓
viremia, with spread to
↓
spleen and liver, where second multiplication occurs, followed by
↓
viremia, with spread to
↓
skin, where development of pox lesions occurs

PICORNA GROUP

The spread of picorna viruses, represented by poliovirus, Coxsackie viruses, and echoviruses, proceeds according to the following diagram. The target organs are in the central nervous system, with varying symptomatology. Multiplication of the virus occurs in lymphoid tissue.

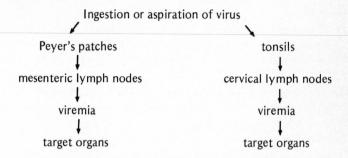

Epidemiology, Diagnosis, and Treatment of Virus Infections

Viral characteristics affecting both epidemiology and treatment are of great importance in dealing with virus infections. Of prime consideration is the fact that virus particles survive in a variety of environmental conditions lethal to most microorganisms. Many viruses are highly resistant to heat, drying, cold, ultraviolet radiation, solvents, and chlorination. In addition, they are noted for mutation, the influenza viruses being especially prone to this process. With mutational capacity in the virus, systematic immunization against the influenza virus is often thwarted; influenza vaccine given in one year may be completely ineffective the next, because the virus has changed its antigenic makeup. The clinical significance of mutation is that people may have repeated episodes of disease due to the same virus. Another important consideration in epidemiology is the sub-clinical case—a fairly common occurrence providing a ready source of infection to the population by means of carriers. Many viral infections do not reach a high enough level of severity to produce overt symptoms, or the symptoms, such as coryza, are too frequently associated with relatively benign diseases.

Diagnosis of virus diseases other than those causing singularly characteristic clinical manifestations, such as pox, is a difficult procedure. There is a common tendency to make a blanket diagnosis of viral infection when otherwise unexplainable symptoms are present. The clinician must be on guard to make a good clinical description of the disease, with accurate recording of the evolution of the signs and symptoms. This is the keystone not only of good clinical medicine but also of good epidemiology and virology.

As in the diagnosis of bacteriologic infection, isolation of the offending organism is the surest means of diagnosis. In viral infections, the sources of material for culture are throat washings, vesicular fluid, feces, or cerebrospinal fluid, the choice of material depending on the virus suspected. Since facilities for virus cultures are not readily available to all clinicians, serologic diagnosis is the best procedure. Even this does have certain limitations in terms of time, since it is not possible to draw solid conclusions on a single, acute-stage serum sample. Rather, paired serums taken during the acute and convalescent stages are necessary, and the interpretation is based on a rise in titer indicated by the convalescent sample. The serologic tests of greatest value are the complement-fixation, neutralizing antibody, and hemagglutination-inhibition tests.

Treatment of viral disease is limited by a similarity between viral resistance to detrimental environmental conditions and their resistance to the currently available antibiotic and chemotherapeutic agents. Treatment, therefore, is largely symptomatic, aside from the possible use, as in measles, of immune γ-globulin, which provides passive immunization.

Varieties of Disease Manifestations (Poliomyelitis)

Poliomyelitis provides a classic example of the range of disease manifestations in virus infection. The outline below indicates the progress of the disease and may be used as a model for many of the diseases caused by the enteroviruses. Polioviruses include three strains: I Brunhilde, II Lansing, and III Leon.

1. Susceptible person is exposed through the upper respiratory tract or contaminated food or water.
2. Within a few hours, mild and transient nasopharyngitis, fever, and headache develop. This is followed by an average 10-day incubation period during which the virus multiplies and spreads.

3. Clinical symptoms of disease develop in varying degrees of severity.

   a. Abortive, or minor, poliomyelitis, with fever, headache, myalgia, and sometimes vomiting.

   b. Nonparalytic, or meningeal, poliomyelitis, with symptoms as in abortive, but with more severe neck and back pain. Cerebrospinal-fluid examination reveals a moderate increase in leukocytes, with lymphocytes predominating. Recovery is rapid and complete.

   c. Paralytic poliomyelitis, with symptoms as in meningeal, but with paralysis related to the site of main attack.

      (1) Spinal, involving motor neurons of the spinal cord.

      (2) Bulbar, involving cranial-nerve nuclei of the medullary center.

      (3) Bulbospinal, involving cranial-nerve nuclei of the medullary center and the motor neurons of the cord, resulting in paralysis of muscles of the extremites, chest, and abdomen.

Vaccine (Poliomyelitis)

The Salk vaccine is made up of killed viruses of all three strains of polio virus and is administered by injection. The viruses used for this vaccine are grown in monkey-kidney tissue culture[1] and inactivated by Formalin. The vaccine is released for use after tests for potency and freedom from bacterial or viral contamination are determined. The Salk vaccine incites a lower level of antibody production than the Sabin preparation does, since the virus particles do not come in contact with the natural sites of invasion and antibody production.

The Sabin vaccine is prepared from organisms cultured in the

[1]Tissue culture is the growing of cells from the body in an artificial medium. The principal tissues so maintained are monkey kidney, amnion, and HeLa cells. HeLa cells (named for the patient from whom they were first obtained) are a propagation of cervical cancer cells. When infected with a virus, the cells in a tissue culture demonstrate cytopathogenic effect by changes in the nucleus and shape of the cell.

same way, but they are live, attenuated organisms. The organisms must be tested for non-neural virulence before the vaccine is released for use. Sabin vaccine is preferred because it is taken by mouth and results in higher antibody titers.

MYCOPLASMA (PPLO)

When first isolated, these organisms were referred to as "pleuro-pneumonia-like organisms"—a term still in common use. They were first found in sputum from patients having atypical pneumonia. They may also be referred to as "Eaton agent" in some of the literature. Their precise place in the taxonomy of microorganisms has not yet been defined, since they have characteristics associated with both viruses and bacteria.

While it is possible to grow *Mycoplasma* on artificial media, the presence of colonies must be determined by microscopic examination and staining of colonies. They are unlike bacteria in that their shape is not consistently defined. They are like viruses in that they can invade living cells and destroy them.

Some *Mycoplasma* are part of the normal flora of the respiratory, intestinal, and genital tracts, causing no disease unless the individual is subjected to unusual stress. For example, cases of puerperal fever have been found to have been caused by this organism.

RICKETTSIA

Named for Howard Taylor Ricketts, who discovered the organism causing Rocky Mountain spotted fever, this group of organisms is considered intermediate between viruses and bacteria. The organisms are obligate parasites, requiring tissue cells for propagation, although the cells need not necessarily be actively metabolizing. The usual culture medium is the yolk sac of embryonated eggs. Patients treated with broad-spectrum antibiotics such as chloromycetin and tetracycline respond well.

Rickettsiae characteristically have their major effect on endothelial cells of the blood vessels. They produce endotoxins similar to those produced by many pathogenic bacteria. Immunity, subsequent to

TABLE 8-2   RICKETTSIAL DISEASES

Disease	Insect vector	Animal reservoir	Locale
Typhus		Rats	United States and
Endemic	Rat flea		Europe
Epidemic	Body louse		
Rocky mountain spotted fever	Tick	Sheep, rodents, dogs	United States and Brazil
Scrub typhus	Akamushi mites	Field mice and other rodents	Japan
Q fever	None	Cattle, sheep	United States and Europe
Rickettsial pox	Mite	House mouse	New York City

SOURCE: After Arthur H. Bryan and Charles G. Bryan, "Bacteriology: Principles and Practice," 3d ed., Barnes & Noble, Inc., New York, 1942, by permission of the publisher.

recovery from an infection, is long-lasting. Certain species of *Rickettsia* show a marked tendency toward latency; i.e., the organism remains in the tissues without causing disease, but recrudesces when the host is subjected to stress.

With the exception of Q fever, rickettsial diseases are spread by insect vectors. The organism of Q fever resists desiccation and is airborne with dust particles contaminated by discharge from infected animals, such as sheep and cattle or man. It is of considerable interest to note that transmission of the insect-borne diseases varies, not always depending on a bite from the insect to infect a new host. For example Rocky Mountain spotted fever can be transmitted by crushing an infected tick on the host's skin. Another important aspect in relation to the persistence of this disease is that an infected tick produces offspring that are infected by way of transovarian transfer. The epidemiology of epidemic typhus is affected by the behavior of the insect vector, the body louse. When the host develops fever, the louse seeks a new host because it is unable to tolerate the host's elevated temperature.

Diagnosis of rickettsial diseases is made by serologic tests based on the fact that antirickettsial antibodies in the serum will agglutinate certain species of the *Proteus* group of bacteria (Weil-Felix reaction).

Complement-fixation tests using rickettsial antigens may also be used. Inoculation of a guinea pig using whole blood from the patient produces characteristic reactions in the scrotal sac when rickettsia are present (Neill-Mooser test).

BACTERIA

Identification

Bacteria are identified by morphology, staining characteristics, biochemical characteristics, and serologic reactions. Smears of material suspected of containing bacteria give information about the type of organism present, thus aiding in the selection of culture media. Cultures further identify the organism by the character of the bacterial colony and the reaction shown in various kinds of media. Serologic reactions then identify the precise species; e.g., enteric bacilli include a number of species with similar staining, morphologic, and cultural characteristics.

MORPHOLOGY

Morphologic identification describes the shape of the organisms: cocci (spheres), bacilli (rods), and spirilliforms (spirals). Cocci include those occurring in pairs (diplococci), in clusters (staphylococci), and in chains (streptococci). Further information may be gained from wet mounts by observating for motility, which indicates a flagellate organism.

STAIN

Staining is essential to classification of bacteria because it makes them easily visible and differentiates various types of organisms by a characteristic kind of stain. Stains may be non-specific (e.g., methylene blue), specific (e.g., Ziehl-Neelsen), and differential (Gram's).

TABLE 8-3   DIFFERENTIAL CHARACTERISTICS
OF COMMON PATHOGENIC BACTERIA

Organism	Gram's stain	Morphology	Other characteristics	Where found
Micrococcus (Staphylo- coccus)	+	Cocci in clusters	Hemolysis; pigment	Ubiquitous
Streptococcus	+	Cocci in chains	Hemolysis (alpha* or beta†)	Throat, sputum, ear, urine, blood, spinal fluid
Corynebacterium diphtheriae	+	Rod, with clubbed ends	Produces toxin	Nasopharynx
Mycobacterium tuberculosis (tubercle bacillus)	+ ‡	Rod	Brittle, yellow colonies	Sputum, pleu- ral fluid, urine, gastric lavage, CSF
Diplococcus pneumoniae	+	Lancet-shaped diplococci	Capsule	Throat, spu- tum, ear, blood, CSF
Clostridium perfringens (welchii) tetani	+	Rod	Spores	Discharge from deep wounds
Neisseria meningitidis	−	Diplococci	Intracellular	CSF, naso- pharynx
Neisseria gonorrhoeae	−	Diplococci	Intracellular	Urethral dis- charge, cer- vical dis- charge, syno- vial fluid
Salmonella typhosa	−	Rod	Nonmotile	Feces; blood in acute stage of typhoid fever
Coliform bacteria	−	Rod	Motile	Intestine; patho- genic in other sites

*Alpha hemolysis produces a greenish color around the colony.
†Beta hemolysis produces a clear zone around the colony.
‡ Gram's stain is not usually used for tubercle bacilli.

TABLE 8-3 (continued)

Organism	Gram's stain	Morphology	Other characteristics	Where found
Salmonella schottmuelleri choleraesuis	—	Rod	Motile	Feces; blood in acute stage of paratyphoid
Pasteurella tularensis	—	Rod		Sputum; ulcer of skin at site of entry
Brucella abortus melitensis suis	—	Rod		Blood; joint spaces
Pseudomonas	—	Rod	Green pigment	Pus from lesions; urine

Specific

Specific stains are for specific organisms. Examples are Albert's stain for diphtheroids and carbolfuchsin solution (Ziehl-Neelsen stain) for the tubercle bacillus. The latter is called an "acid-fast" organism because it retains the red color of the carbolfuchsin dye despite treatment with acid alcohol to remove the stain. Non-acid-fast material loses the red color and is visualized by a counterstain of some other color, such as methylene blue.

Differential

The differential, or Gram's, stain combines two stains, gentian violet and safranin. Gram's stain differentiates bacteria into two classes: those which stain purple (gram-positive) and those which stain red (gram-negative).

PREPARATION OF SMEARS

Although smears from the material or swabs brought to the bacteriologist are ordinarily prepared by the laboratory, there are occasions when others may be called upon to prepare them. The following points to remember in preparing smears will ensure good results and aid the bacteriologist:

1. Clean, nongreasy slides are essential. It is desirable to have new slides for this work, although previously used slides can be used again if they are not scratched.
2. Gently spread the material on an area near the center of the slide, making it neither too thick nor too thin. When the material is sparse, do not spread it over a wide area but outline the area containing the material with a glass-marking pencil on the *underside* of the slide.
3. In smears for gonococci, *roll* rather than rub the swab on the slide and do not cover the same area twice.
4. Attach proper identification of patient and source of smear.

COLLECTION OF MATERIAL FOR BACTERIAL CULTURES

The cardinal rule is to avoid contamination of the area involved in the infectious process and to obtain truly representative material. For example, collecting material from skin lesions requires that the area be cleaned with alcohol before pus is taken from the lesion and that the material be obtained from well within the lesion rather than superficially, since skin normally has bacteria present. Correct identification of the patient, source of material, and disease suspected is essential to the investigation of a bacterial disease. Material from exudates of the nose, nasopharynx, and tonsils should be obtained on two swabs. When Vincent's angina (trench mouth) is suspected, only smears are needed for diagnosis.

Urine (Routine)

Method of collection. Specimens are collected from women as follows:

1. Clean the entire vulvar area with soap and water followed by Zephiran Chloride (1:1,000).

2. Have the patient hold the labia apart and, after passing some urine, void directly into the sterile bottle, collecting the midstream portion of the voiding.
3. Cap the bottle with a sterile cap and take it directly to the laboratory. Note the method of collection of all specimens for urine culture.

Catheterization may be necessary in some cases. Clean-voided specimens are preferred, however, since contamination of the bladder results in a significant percentage of cases in which catheterization was done. As has been noted, it is less objectionable to contaminate the urine specimen than the bladder.

Specimens are collected from men as follows:

1. Clean the meatus and surrounding parts well with soap and water followed by Zephiran Chloride (1:1,000).
2. Have the patient, after passing some urine, void directly into the sterile bottle, collecting the midstream portion of the voiding.
3. Cap the bottle with a sterile cap and take it directly to the laboratory.

Quantitative urine culture. With the use of clean-voided specimens for urine cultures, it is necessary to know the number of organisms per milliliter of specimen in order to interpret the results accurately. This is why it is of utmost importance to the microbiologist to know the method used in collecting the specimen.

For a quantitative culture, the microbiologist inoculates a specific amount of specimen on three plates, one with the undiluted sample (if the urine is clear) and the other two plates with different dilutions. After suitable incubation, the number of colonies is counted on the plate showing the fewest colonies and multiplied by the appropriate dilution factor to determine the number of organisms per milliliter. A count of 10,000 or less is considered due to transurethral or external contamination. A count of 50,000 to 100,000 represents probably infection, and more than 100,000 represents definite infection. The organism(s) causing the infection are are then identified, and sensitivity are tests done.

The organisms which are found most frequently in urinary-tract infections are *E. coli, Aerobacter aerogenes, Pseudomonas aeruginosa, Proteus, Alcaligenes fecalis, Staphylococcus,* and certain strains of *Streptococcus.*

Urine for Tubercle Bacilli

A first morning specimen (preferably catheterized, since acid-fast saprophytes are common to the urethral area) is collected in a sterile bottle. The specimen, labeled with the request for TB culture, is taken directly to the laboratory.

Gastric Lavage for Tubercle Bacilli

Gastric lavage is necessary in patients who do not raise sputum, in order to confirm diagnosis of tuberculosis. With the patient in the fasting state, sterile distilled water is introduced into the stomach after passage of a clean Levin tube in the usual manner. The water is then removed by aspiration and placed in a sterile flask. The specimen should be treated to neutralize the acid if it must await the attention of the bacteriologist more than 1 h.

Sputum

Sputum specimens for detection of the type of organism causing pneumonia should be collected in a petri dish or a sputum cup. The specimen may be collected at any time when the patient is able to raise material from his lungs. If delay in delivering the sample to the laboratory or in starting the culture is unavoidable, the sample should be refrigerated to avoid overgrowth of nonpathogenic bacteria which are present. The patient must be careful to avoid contaminating the outside of the container.

In cases of known or suspected tuberculosis, 24-h samples of sputum are recommended. They are collected in a sterile bottle. Again, it is imperative that the patient be instructed to avoid contamination of the outside of the bottle.

Blood

Ordinarily, laboratory personnel collect blood for cultures. The venipuncture site is cleaned with alcohol, the skin is cleaned with Merthiolate, and the venipuncture is performed. The technologist obtains blood in a sterile syringe and inoculates the various media for blood culture directly. Sterile Vacutainer tubes may also be used to collect the sample.

Vaginal and Cervical Material

If gonorrhea is suspected, two swabs of material are required: one for the smear and one for the culture. When delay in delivery to the laboratory is unavoidable, the swab for culture should be placed in a tube of special transport medium. If trichomoniasis is suspected, the material should be placed in a small amount of saline solution and examined immediately.

Stools

Stool cultures for bacterial or viral agents require only a small amount of feces; therefore it is unnecessary to send the entire specimen to the laboratory for this purpose. With diarrheal stools, a large cotton swab dipped in the specimen (particularly in purulent-appearing masses) is quite satisfactory for culture. In bacillary dysentery, rectal swabs are a simple and satisfactory means of obtaining material. The anus is kept patent by insertion of a tube, through which a long cotton swab is inserted and material obtained from the rectum. The swab is then placed in a sterile test tube for delivery to the laboratory.

BACTERIOPHAGE TYPING

With the concern about epidemics of staphylococcus infections, there is a need to know the precise type of staphylococcus involved in any cases of epidemic infection. This is accomplished by inoculating known bacteriophages (viruses parasitic to specific species of bacteria) with cultures of staphylococci and observing for plaques. Plaques are areas of lysis of the organisms. The investigation is also referred to as "phage" typing.

Sensitivity of Bacteria to Antibiotics

In addition to identifying the organism causing infection, it is helpful to know which antibiotic is most effective against it. For this purpose, the isolated organism is streaked heavily on agar plates, and paper disks impregnated with known concentrations of each antibiotic are placed on the surface. The plate is then incubated the proper length of time. Inhibition of growth ground the disks is indicative of the organisms's sensitivity to the given antibiotic. Another, though more laborious, method is to inoculate the organism into broths containing known amounts of antibiotics and then to note inhibition of growth. For the proper handling of culture materials, the technologist must know which, if any, antibiotics the patient may be receiving at the time the specimen is collected. To test for the antibiotic level in the patient's serum, serial dilutions are made, and the organism is inoculated in each tube. After incubation, the tubes are inspected for growth, and the titer is reported.

Bacterial Toxins

The severity of many of the infectious diseases depends upon their adversely affecting the tissue invaded, but a significant number of organisms produce serious disease because of the effect of their toxins. Endotoxins are substances that are found in the cell walls of bacteria; they are common to most bacteria and are unquestionably contributors to the general disease process. Exotoxins are substances that are secreted by bacteria; only a few bacterial groups produce exotoxins. Table 8-4 shows a comparison of the properties associated with endo- and exotoxins. As is shown in Table 8-5, even within a single genus of exotoxin-producing organisms there are differences in specificity.

One of the better-known exotoxin-producing organisms is the

TABLE 8-4   COMPARISON OF ENDOTOXIN AND EXOTOXIN

Characteristic	Endotoxin	Exotoxin
Diffusion from bacterial cell	0	+
Potency	++	++++
Antigenicity	+	++++
Reaction to heat	Stable	Labile
Tissue action	Nonspecific	Selective
Chemical composition	Protein or glucolipoid	Protein
Destruction by proteolytic enzymes	0	+
Detoxication by Formalin	0	+
Source	Most organisms pathogenic to man	Clostridia, C. diphtheriae, Shigella dysenteriae

virulent strain of *Corynebacterium diphtheriae*. It has been found that the virulence (i.e., ability to synthesize toxin) is dependent upon prior bacteriophage infection of the diphtheria organism and the iron content of the medium in which it grows. When diphtherial organisms are isolated in culture, a virulence test must be done in order to identify them as virulent, pathogenic strains.

SPIRELLA AND SPIROCHETES

These organisms are, as their names indicate, spiral in form. Most of the spirella organisms may be cultured, but there is no practical means of culturing the spirochetes. Serologic diagnosis of spirochete diseases is necessary, although dark-field microscopic examination of lesions produced by the spirochetes may be used. As noted in Table 8-6, yaws and syphilis are the spirochetal diseases. The spirella diseases are characterized by marked fever (with the exception of *B. vincentii*).

FUNGI AND YEASTS

Mycotic infections are serious because of their resistance to treatment by the usual means. Fungi are plants. Fungi of medical interest

TABLE 8-5 COMPARISONS IN THE GENUS *Clostridium*

Characteristics	*Cl. tetani*	*Cl. perfringens*	*Cl. botulinum*
Type of toxin	Neurotoxin	Tissue toxin	Neurotoxin
Dose lethal to laboratory animals*	6×10^{-6}		4.5×10^{-9}
Symptoms	Spastic paralysis of voluntary muscles	Tissue necrosis with crepitation; foul smell; shock; collapse; death	Inability to focus eyes well; flaccid paralysis of chest muscles
Treatment	Prophylaxis in any puncture wound;† cleansing and debridement; antitoxin in large doses; avoidance of any stimulation to prevent convulsions; penicillin	Debridement of contaminated and devitalized tissue (amputation of an affected extremity may be necessary); penicillin	Large doses of antitoxin early in the disease (must be of the specific type A, B, or E)
Prophylaxis	Immunization with tetanus toxoid	None routinely done	Not done; best prevention is to boil home-canned foods 10 min to inactivate toxin

*Measures of toxic doses are in milligrams of nitrogen contained in the toxin molecule.

†If the antitoxin is derived from horse serum, it is imperative that a skin test for sensitivity to the serum be done in order to avoid hypersensitive allergic reaction.

are those which produce diseases of the skin (superficial mycoses) and internal organs (deep, or systemic, mycoses). Diagnosis depends upon isolation of the fungus and, in some cases, skin tests or serologic tests.

TABLE 8-6   SPIRELLA AND SPIROCHETE DISEASES

Organism	Disease	Mode of transmission	Morphology of coils	Diagnostic material
Spirella				
Borrelia re currentis	European relapsing fever	Human body louse	Loose	Blood smear at onset of relapse; culture
B. novyi	American relapsing fever	Ticks	Loose	Blood smear at onset of relapse; culture
B. vincentii	Vincent's angina (trench mouth)	Contact	Loose	Smear from lesion (fusiform bacilli also seen)
Leptospira icterohaemorrhagiae	Well's disease (infectious jaundice)	Rat to man	Tight, with hooked ends	Blood smear; culture
L. canicola	Canicola fever	Dog to man	Tight, with hooked ends	Blood smear; culture
Spirillum minus	Rat-bite fever	Rat to man	Short, thick	Blood smear; guinea pig inoculation
Spirochetes				
Treponema pallidum	Syphilis	Contact	Tight	Chancre fluid; serum for STS
T. pertenue	Yaws	Contact; fly bite	Tight	Lesion fluid; serum for STS

SOURCE: From Israel Davidsohn and John B. Henry (eds.), "Todd-Sanford Clinical Diagnosis by Laboratory Methods," 15th ed., p. 997, W. B. Saunders Company, Philadelphia, 1974.

In the superficial mycoses, it is necessary to obtain material from within the lesion or small bits or tissue, such as nails, skin, or hair, depending on the location of the infection. In the deep mycoses, smears and cultures of material obtained from the lesions (such as sputum for pulmonary mysosis) are important for diagnosis.

TABLE 8-7   MYCOTIC INFECTIONS

Organism	Diseases	Type of involvement	Material studied
Superficial			
Microsporum	Dermatomycoses,	Usually primarily	Hair, nails, and
Trichophyton	ringworm, favus	cutaneous	skin scrapings
Epidermophyton		lesions, with	
Achorion		pus and no definite systemic disease	
Superficial or systemic			
Monilia	Thrush; ulcerative,	Usually primarily	Scrapings from
Blastomyces	exfoliative,	mucous-membrane	skin, if superficial; sputum,
Coccidioides	suppurative,	and skin	if systemic
Sporotrichum	and vesicular types of dermatitis	infection, with frequent systemic disease	
Systemic			
Cryptococcus (Torula)	Cerebral and pulmonary granulomas	Primary system-disease	CSF, sputum
Aspergillus	Otomycosis and focal pulmonary lesions	Primary systemic disease; may be seen in skin or mucous-membrane infection	Sputum
Histoplasma	Pulmonary	Primary systemic disease	Sputum

SOURCE: After Arthur H. Bryan and Charles G. Bryan, "Bacteriology: Principles and Practice," 3d ed., Barnes & Noble, Inc., New York, 1942, by permission of the publisher.

ANIMAL PARASITES

Parasites to which man is subject include a wide range of animals from the microscopic protozoans to relatively large organisms. With even the most remote regions of the world easily accessible to travel, the incidence of so-called exotic parasitic diseases, once considered to be confined to certain regions, is rising. It must be remembered that, although the patient's symptoms of parasitic infection might not develop until he has returned to his home, the possibility of a disease common in another region is a real one. In addition, animal reservoirs of these regional diseases may be brought to other areas. For example, a case has been reported of schistosomiasis which the patient contracted from tending an aquarium in which the snail which harbors the larval forms of *Schistosoma haematobium* was present.

Rather than a detailed description of the complicated life cycles of parasites found in man, the material in Table 8-8 shows only those portions involved in the transfer of the organism from non-human to human hosts. Choice of material for diagnosis depends upon knowledge of life cycles. In addition, in the efforts toward control and eradication of parasitic diseases, it is important to know the most vulnerable point in the life cycle of a given parasite so that control measures can be applied most effectively and economically. Thus, in the case of malaria, control of the mosquito population is the procedure of choice. It is important to know the portion of the life cycle during which infection takes place in order to protect oneself and others and to instruct patients. Figure 8-1 shows the five types of life cycles known in the transmission of parasitic infection from animal (or man) to man.

Intestinal Parasites

Diagnosis of intestinal parasites is made upon finding in the stool either the parasite itself in trophozoic (active, adult) or cystic form or upon finding the ova characteristic of the animal. Specimens are collected in the following manner:

1. *Loose, fluid stools.* These stools are likely to show the tropho-

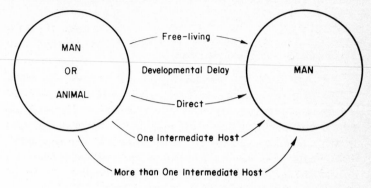

FIG. 8-1 Typical animal parasite transmission.

zoites of the intestinal amoebas and flagellates. These stools must be kept at body temperature and examined within 30 min of collection if the organisms are to be found in the active state. A simple method of maintaining the temperature is to place the container holding the specimen in a pan of warm water.

2. *Well-formed or semiformed stools.* These stools contain ova or the cystic forms of parasites, neither of which require the maintenance of body temperature. They do not need to be kept warm or examined as immediately.

3. Treatment for tapeworms is not complete unless the scolex (head) of the parasite is discharged from the intestine. Consequently, after medication to dislodge the scolex has been administered, a purgative is given and *all resulting stools* are examined *in their entirety* to find the scolex.

4. Since the habitat of the pinworm is the lower intestinal tract and the femal pinworm migrates to the anus to discharge the ova, particularly at night, a satisfactory means of diagnosing this type of infestation is the cellophane-tape slide. A piece of cellophane tape is placed across the anus, removed immediately, and stuck on an ordinary slide. Microscopic examination of the slide will reveal the ova of this parasite adhered to the tape. Positive examinations are more likely to result from preparations made

from early morning specimens, obtained before the patient has gone to stool or dressed.

Toxoplasma gondii (Toxoplasmosis)

Although toxoplasmosis in adults (acquired) is not usually serious, a critical aspect of the disease is the possibility of congenital infection, with a variety of pathologic effects including encephalitis. In adults, some of the findings, such as atypical lymphocytes, tend to resemble infectious mononucleosis when associated with lymphadeopathy. Cats have been implicated as the animal reservoir for *Toxoplasma.*

INSECTS ASSOCIATED WITH DISEASE

Insects that live on the surface of the human body are called *ectoparasites.* Insects that transmit pathogenic organisms to other animals, including man, are called *insect vectors.* Some ectoparasites are also insect vectors; however, many insect vectors spread disease through only transitory contact with the host or the host's food.

Ectoparasites

ITCH MITE

The well-known "itch mite," *Sarcoptes scabiei,* causes scabies. It is diagnosed by finding the insect's burrow in the skin, with the aid of a magnifying glass, and by examining scrapings from the suspected area for eggs of the parasite.

LICE

Three species of lice are parasitic to man, and each makes its habitat in different regions of the body.

1. *Pediculus humanus* var. *capitis* is the head louse and is diagnosed by examining hairs for the presence of eggs (nits) and adult insects.

2. *Pediculus humanus* var. *corporis* is the body louse, which lives in the clothing and attaches itself to the body only when feeding. Its eggs are found in the folds and seams of clothing.
3. *Phthirius pubis* is the pubic louse and is found on the hairs of the pubic area. As with the head louse, diagnosis is made by examining hairs for the presence of eggs.

TICKS

These ectoparasites are known to be vectors of spirella, rickettsia, viruses, and some bacteria. They may be hard-bodied or soft-bodied, depending on the presence or absence of a dorsal plate. The tick integument is characteristically leathery. Ticks are common ectoparasites on animals, some of which may be reservoirs for infectious organisms.

Transitory Insects

BEDBUGS

Cimex lectularius, the bedbug, lives primarily in furniture, floors, and walls. It feeds on the human body at night. It may transmit bacteria incidentally. The infection of the bite is secondary to scratching the site.

FLIES

Bloodsucking flies are important as insect vectors. The nonbloodsucking flies, such as *Musca domestica* (common housefly), may transmit disease incidentally. Larvae hatched from eggs of these flies deposited in wounds or sores are, in effect, parasites, causing myiasis.

MOSQUITOES

Mosquitoes are in the fly family. They are vectors of some virus diseases and of filariasis, and they are hosts as well as vectors in the malarial-parasite life cycles.

TABLE 8-8 PARASITES

Organism	Common name or disease	Habitat in man	Diagnostic material	Route of infection	Ineffective stage
Endamoeba histolytica	Amoebiasis	Intestine, liver abscess	Stool for trophozoic or cyctic forms	Ingestion of cysts in contaminated water or food	Cysts
Trichomonas vaginalis		Female genital tract, male urethra	Discharge (for hanging drop prep.)	Direct contact	Trophozoites
Plasmodium	Malaria	1–3. Erythrocytes	1–3. Blood	1–3. Bite of *Anopheles* mosquito, blood transfusion	1–3. Micro-gametes and macrogam-metes from mosquito; schizonts or gametes from blood trans-fusion
1. *P. vivax*	1. Tertian malaria				
2. *P. malariae*	2. Quartan malaria				
3. *P. falciparum*	3. Malignant tertian				
Leishmania					
1. *L. donovanii*	1. Kala-azar	1. Reticuloendo-thelial system	1. Blood, bone marrow	1–3. Bite of sandfly (*Phlebotomus*)	1–3. Leish-monads
2. *L. tropica*	2. Oriental sore	2. Skin	2. Skin scrap-ings		

			3. Material from lesions		
3. *L. brasiliensis*	3. Forest yaws	3. Mucocutaneous area of nose, mouth, pharynx			
Trypanosoma 1. *T. gambiense* 2. *T. rhodesiense*	1-2. African sleeping sickness	Blood, lymph glands, brain	1-2. Blood	1-2. Bite of tsetse fly	1-3. Meta-cyclic form
3. *T. cruzi*	3. Chagas' disease		3. Blood culture, complement-fixation test	3. Bite of *Triatoma* (kissing bug) infected by the insect's feces	
Loa loa	Eye worm	Subcutaneous tissue	Blood (during the day) for larval forms	Bite of the deer fly	Filariform larvae
Wuchereria bancrofti	Filariasis, elephantiasis	Lymph nodes (adults), blood (larvae)	Blood for larval forms	Bite of *Culex* or *Aedes* mosquito	Filariform larvae
Onchocerca volvulus		Subcutaneous connective tissue	Biopsy	Bite of the black gnat or jinja fly	Filariform larvae
Strongyloides stercoralis	Threadworm	Intestine	Stool for adult worms	Larvae in contaminated soil penetrate skin	Filariform larvae
Ancylostoma duodenale *Necator americanus*	Old World hookworm New World hookworm	Intestine	Stool for ova and adults	Larvae in contaminated soil penetrate skin	Filariform larvae

TABLE 8-8 (continued)

Organism	Common name or disease	Habitat in man	Diagnostic material	Route of infection	Ineffective stage
Ascaris lumbricoides	Roundworm	Intestine	Stool for ova	Ingestion of embryonated ova	Ova after 10–14 days incubation in warm soil
Trichuris trichiria	Whipworm	Intestine	Stool for ova	Ingestion of embryonated ova	Ova after suitable incubation in warm moist soil
Enterobius vermicularis	Pinworm	Intestine	Cellophane-tape "smear"	Ingestion of ova	Ova immediately infective on discharge from the body
Trichinella spiralis		Intestine (adult), striated muscle (cyst)	Biopsy, skin test	Eating undercooked pork	Cysts in contaminated pork
Fasciolopsis buski	Intestinal fluke	Intestine	Stool for ova	Eating contaminated water chestnuts	Larvae encysted on water chestnuts
Paragonimus westermani	Lung fluke	Lung	Sputum or stool for ova	Eating undercooked crab or crayfish	Larvae in intermediate hosts
Clonorchis sinensis	Liver fluke	Liver	Stool for ova	Eating undercooked fish	Larval cysts in fish

Organism	Common name	Location	Specimen	Source of infection	Infective form
Schistosoma					
1. *S. hematobium*	1–3. Blood fluke	1. Venous plexus of urinary bladder	1. Urine for ova	Contact with contaminated water	Cercariae in water penetrate the skin
2. *S. mansoni*		2. Venous plexus of colon	2–3. Stool for ova		
3. *S. japonicum*		3. Venous plexus of small intestine			
Dracunculus medinensis	Skin ulcer	Skin, subcutaneous tissue	Contents of vesicle	Drinking water contaminated with *Cyclops*	Larvae in the crustacean *Cyclops*
Taenia					
1. *T. saginata*	1. Beef tapeworm	Intestine	Stool for ova, proglottids, scolex	1. Eating undercooked beef	1. Larval cysts in beef
2. *T. solium*	2. Pork tapeworm			2. Eating undercooked pork	2. Larval cysts in pork
Diphyllobothrium latium	Fish tapeworm	Intestine	Stool for ova proglottids, scolex	Eating undercooked fish	Larval cysts in fish
Hymenolepsis nana	Dwarf tapeworm	Intestine	Stool for ova, proglottids, scolex	Ingestion of fertile ova	Ova after several hours incubation following discharge from bowel
Echinococcus granulosus	Dog tapeworm, hydatid cyst	Intestine (adult), internal organs (cyst)	Aspiration of cyst contents, skin test	Ingestion of ova	Ova in contaminated soil

REFERENCES

"Atlas of Diagnostic Microbiology," Abbott Laboratories, North Chicago, Ill., 1966.

Bailey, W., and E. G. Scott: "Diagnostic Microbiology," 3d ed., Mosby, St. Louis, 1970.

Belding, David L.: "Textbook of Parasitology," 3d ed., Appleton-Century-Crofts, New York, 1965.

Beneke, E. S., and A. L. Rogers: "Medical Mycology Manual," 3d ed., Burgess, Minneapolis, 1971.

Bodily, H. L., et al.: "Diagnostic Procedures for Bacterial, Mycotic, and Parasitic Infections," 5th ed., American Public Health Association, New York, 1970.

Davidsohn, Israel, and John B. Henry (eds.): "Todd-Sanford Clinical Diagnosis by Laboratory Methods," 15th ed., Saunders, Philadelphia, 1974.

Dubos, Rene (ed.): "Bacterial and Mycotic Infections of Man," 4th ed., Lippincott, Philadelphia, 1969.

Emmons, C. W., C. H. Binford, and J. P. Utz: "Medical Mycology," 2d ed., Lea & Febiger, Philadelphia, 1970.

Faust, E. C., P. R. Russell, and R. C. Jung: "Craig-Faust Clinical Parasitology," 8th ed., Lea & Febiger, Philadelphia, 1970.

Ginsberg, Marian K., and Maria Laconte: Reverse Isolation, *Am. J. Nurs.*, **64**(9):88, 1964.

Graber, C. D.: "Rapid Daignostic Methods in Medical Microbiology," Williams & Wilkins, Baltimore, 1970.

Haley, L.: "Diagnostic Medical Mycology," Appleton-Century-Crofts, New York, 1964.

Hedgecock, Loyd: "Antimicrobial Agents," Lea & Febiger, Philadelphia, 1967.

Horsfal, F. L., and I. Tamm (eds.): "Viral and Rickettsial Diseases of Man" 4th ed., Lippincott, Philadelphia, 1965.

"Infection Control in the Hospital," American Hospital Association, Chicago, 1970.

Jansson, E.: Isolation of Fastidious Mycoplasma from Human Sources, *J. Clin. Path.*, **24**:253, 1971.

Lennette, E. H., and N. J. Schmidt (eds.): "Diagnostic Procedures in Viral and Rickettsial Infections," 4th ed., American Public Health Association, New York, 1969.

Markell, E. K., and M. Voge: "Medical Parasitology," 3d ed., Saunders, Philadelphia, 1971.

McQuay, R. M.: Good Parasitology Examinations Depend on Proper Procedures, *Hosp. Top.*, **44**:85, 1966.

"Principles and Practice of Autoclave Sterilization," Aseptic-Thermo Indicator Co., North Hollywood, Calif., 1965.

"Principles of Asepsis," American Nurses Association, New York, 1964.

Rebell, G., and D. Taplin: "Dermatophytes. Their Recognition and Identification," 2d ed., University of Miami Press, Coral Gables, Fla., 1970.

Snyder, J. E.: Infection Control, *Hospitals*, **44**:58, 1970.

Stuart, R. D.: Transport Media for Specimens in Public Health Bacteriology, *Public Health Rep.*, **74**:431, 1959.

NINE

CEREBROSPINAL-FLUID EXAMINATIONS

GENERAL CONSIDERATIONS

The cerebrospinal fluid (CSF) is the near equivalent of tissue fluid in other parts of the body. Normally it is a clear, colorless fluid. It is the product of filtration and secretion of the cells of the choroid plexus. It circulates over the brain and into the spinal canal. The normal total volume is about 1.5 dl. It functions to maintain optimal intracranial pressure and to protect the central nervous system. The normal pressure of the CSF is 7 to 10 mm Hg when the patient is in a horizontal position.

CSF is obtained by introducing a needle into the spinal canal. The usual site of the puncture is the lumbar area. The patient lies on his side with his knees drawn up sufficiently to bow the back somewhat. When the spinal canal is entered, the physician tests the pressure with a manometer and then allows the fluid to drip into a series of small sterile test tubes, collecting 2 to 3 ml fluid in each of at least three tubes, which are numbered in sequence of collection. Even though no apparent trauma may have occurred during the puncture, it is possible to rupture a very small blood vessel in the process, contaminating the fluid with a small amount of blood. Since the presence of blood alters the level of normal constituents of CSF, it is important to flush the needle with fluid (tube 1) and examine the uncontaminated fluid (tubes 2 and 3).

The lumbar puncture is not too painful a procedure for the patient. However, because of the reduced volume of CSF, the patient may note headache if he is upright immediately after the procedure. It is advisable, therefore, for the patient to lie flat for a while until equilibrium can be reestablished.

EXAMINATIONS OF CEREBROSPINAL FLUID

The cardinal rule for examining CSF is that it be done as quickly as possible after obtaining the specimen. This is particularly true of cell counts and bacterial examinations.

Gross Appearance

A description of the gross appearance of the fluid is part of the report. This includes color and degree of cloudiness, if any, or the presence of frank blood. Xanthochromia, or yellow coloration, of the CFS is most frequently due to the breakdown of red blood cells in the cerebrospinal system. When the CFS is bloody, to rule out the possibility of traumatic tap, the fluid is inspected after the cells are removed by centrifugation, and the yellow color is revealed if the blood is not due to trauma of tap. Severe jaundice, metastatic melanoma, Weil's disease, and very high protein levels are other conditions that also will yield xanthochromic CFS.

Chemical Examination

GLUCOSE

Glucose levels in CSF are influenced by the concentration of glucose in the blood, since CFS contains a number of blood constituents. It is also necessary, therefore, to obtain a blood glucose determination in order to interpret the results of the CSF determination precisely. The normal level for CFS glucose is 60 to 80 percent of the blood glucose level.

PROTEINS

Proteins are normally present in relatively low concentrations, ranging between 20 and 40 mg/dl CSF, with 50 to 70 percent in the albumin fraction. An increase in the amount of protein indicates irritation of the meninges, as in inflammatory processes, or spinal block because of a tumor. Tests such as the Pandy, Nonne-Apelt, or zinc sulfate turbidity are semiquantitative and are, at best, only rough screening tests. Quantitative tests for proteins should be used to assist in more definitive diagnoses. CSF protein electrophoresis is a useful means of determining the percent of the total protein fractions. Unless the total protein is elevated significantly, it is advisable to use a concentrate made from 10 to 15 ml CSF for accurate electrophoresis. The macroglobulin of multiple myeloma is readily identified by electrophoresis. It is possible for the globulin fraction to be elevated even when the total protein is within normal limits. As a rule, the globulin is increased in relation to the total protein.

Microscopic Examination

CELL COUNTS

Cell counts are done with the instruments that are used for blood counts. It is necessary to make cell counts quickly because the cells tend to clump on standing, thus yielding erroneous results. In cell counts of significant levels, a differential count is done, in addition to the total count, in order to give additional information as to the type of inflammatory process present.

BACTERIAL SMEAR AND CULTURES

Smears and cultures for bacteria are absolutely essential in any case of suspected meningitis. Reports from smears can mean the difference between life and death, and they are therefore done as quickly as possible in order that treatment may be instituted without delay. Since the meningitic infections are usually caused by a highly virulent organism, special care must be taken to avoid self-contamination with the material.

Serologic Examination

A positive serologic test for syphilis usually is interpreted to indicate involvement of the central servous system in the disease process. It should be noted that positive CSF results are not an indication that the disease is active, for even after syphilis has been adequately treated, positive CSF results may be obtained. The VDRL flocculation test for syphilis is the most common procedure used.

The Lange colloidal gold test is done by adding a colloidal suspension of a gold salt to serially diluted CSF and observing for color changes. The changes are the result of the breakdown of the colloidal state of the gold salt. Globulin is believed to influence precipitation of the salt. Results are reported according to color changes in each of the ten tubes used in the serial dilutions, as follows; 0 = red, 1 = reddish-blue, 2 = purple, 3 = deep blue, 4 = light blue, 5 = colorless. Sample colloidal gold test results are given below:

Normal: 0-0-0-0-0-0-0-0-0-0 or 0-0-0-1-2-1-0-0-0-0
Suggestive of multiple sclerosis: 5-5-5-5-4-2-1-0-0-0
CNS syphilis: 0-1-2-3-1-0-0-0-0-0- or 5-5-5-5-5-4-2-1-0-0

In the absence of a positive STS, a positive colloidal gold is suggestive of multiple sclerosis. CSF electrophoresis studies are helpful in differential diagnosis of multiple sclerosis.

TABLE 9-1   SOME TYPICAL CSF FINDINGS

Condition	WBC	Total Protein	Glucose
Normal	0–5	20–40 mg/dl	60–80% of blood level
Bacterial infection	200 or more*	Elevated	Decreased
Viral infection	100 or more†	Normal to slightly elevated	Normal
Tuberculous infection	50–100†	Usually elevated	Decreased
CNS syphilis	10–60†	Normal to slightly elevated	Normal
Multiple sclerosis	0–5	Normal to slightly elevated	Normal

*Predominantly neutrophils.
†Predominantly lymphocytes.

REFERENCES

Cole, M.: Pitfalls in Cerebrospinal Fluid Examination, *Hosp. Pract.*, 4:47, 1969.

Davidsohn, Israel, and John B. Henry (eds.): "Todd-Sanford Clinical Diagnosis by Laboratory Methods," 15th ed., Saunders, Philadelphia, 1975.

Green, J. B.: The Colloidal Gold Test of the Spinal Fluid, *JAMA*, 209:1908, 1969.

Kaplan, A.: Electrophoresis of Cerebrospinal Fluid Proteins, *Amer. J. Med. Sci.*, 253:549, 1967.

Windisch, R. M., and M. M. Bracken: Cerebrospinal Fluid Proteins: Concentration by Membrane Ultrafiltration and Fractionation by Electrophoresis on Cellulose Acetate, *Clin. Chem.*, 16:415, 1970.

TEN

MISCELLANEOUS EXAMINATIONS

HISTOLOGIC EXAMINATIONS

General Considerations

The microscopic examination of tissue is a cornerstone of diagnosis, for it is, in many cases, the most definitive form of diagnosis. Since the cells and their relationship to one another are the basis of this type of examination, the first consideration must be preserving the cells as near to the living state as possible. It is frequently the nurse who deals first with the tissues removed for biopsy examination or extirpation. Understanding the reasons for what she does should make it easier for her to execute this first step in histologic examinations and to aid the pathologist in his task.

Fixation of Tissues

Fixation refers to arresting the life process in the tissue cells. It is accomplished by coagulating the proteins of the cells and halting enzymatic activity by chemical means. The usual solutions used to fix tissues are 80% alcohol and 10% Formalin. Other solutions may be used for special analyses of tissue enzymes or other cellular constituents, and in such cases the laboratory supplies the material and instructions.

The recommended proportion of specimen and fixative is an amount of fixative solution 10 times the volume of the specimen. It is important that the specimen be immersed completely in the solution as soon as possible in order to prevent dehydration, bacterial growth, and enzymatic activity, all of which alter the structure and relationships of the cells of the tissue.

Frozen Sections

For quick diagnosis of possible malignant lesions, the frozen section is the best procedure. Rather than being processed in the usual way, the specimen is quick-frozen, cut, and stained immediately. Although this method is valuable because it is quick, the sections prepared in this manner are not satisfactory for detailed study of the cells, and they are not permanent. Additional sections are usually prepared in the standard manner for study at leisure.

EXFOLIATIVE CYTOLOGY

Developed by Dr. George Papanicolaou primarily for the diagnosis of early cervical malignant conditions, the technique of exfoliative cytology has grown to include many areas. The term *exfoliative cytology* means the study of cells that have sloughed off. This is a natural event in both normal and malignant epithelial tissues. By studying cells of this type, one can frequently diagnose malignant conditions before the lesion has advanced to the stage at which overt symptoms are noticed by the patient. A positive

Papanicolaou smear is always followed by biopsy to confirm the diagnosis before further treatment is instituted.

The following types of material are suitable for Papanicolaou stains:

1. Cervical secretions
2. Bronchial secretions and washings
3. Urine sediment
4. Pleural- and peritoneal-fluid sediment
5. Mammary gland discharge fluid

To ensure maximal accuracy in Papanicolaou smears, material should be treated according to the following instructions:

1. Fix the specimen (smear) by immersing the slide in a fixative solution of equal parts of ether and 95% ethyl alcohol.
2. Remove the slide after 30 min in the fixative solution, allow it to dry, and send it to the cytotechnologist or pathologist for staining and analysis.
3. When materials are not immediately smeared, send the specimen containing the cells (e.g., urine) to the laboratory immediately, where the proper fixation, etc. will be done.

Papanicolaou smears are reported in a five-point scale as follows:

Grade I.   Absence of atypical or abnormal cells
Grade II.   Atypical cytology but no evidence of malignancy
Grade III. Cytology suggests, but is not conclusive for, malignancy
Grade IV.   Strongly suggestive of malignancy
Grade V.   Conclusive for malignancy

ELECTROCARDIOGRAM

The electrocardiogram (EKG or ECG) constitutes a "picture" of the heartbeat. Electrodes are attached to each limb and to the precordium, and a portrait of the heart action is obtained from various combinations of the electrodes. The electric impulses generated by the heart as part of its action are picked up by the electrodes and magnified by passage through vacuum tubes and thence to a galvanometer, which is deflected within a magnetic field in accordance with the charge of the impulses. The deflections of the galvanometer are produced by positive and negative charges and are recorded on a special paper or photographic film. Rhythm, site of the pacemaker, position of the heart, size of the ventricles, and presence of injury currents are revealed by the electrocardiographic tracing.

The pacemaker in the normal heart action is the sinus node, which is located on the right atrium. The node is a very small bundle of modified muscle tissue which discharges an electric impulse rhythmically and thus initiates the heart action. The electric charge spreads through the whole mass of atrial tissue because the muscle fibers are connected by protoplasmic bridges. The electric impulse is carried to the atrioventricular (AV) node and thence throughout the ventricular tissue, completing the route and causing the ventricles to contract as did the atria when they were subject to the electric excitation. Figure 10-1 shows the pattern produced by the electrocardiogram as the heart action takes place.

Each combination of electrodes used in the standard electrocardiogram is called a *lead*. Lead I is the electrodes attached to the arms; lead II is the right-arm—left-leg combination; and lead III is the left-arm—left-leg combination. For the chest, or precordial, leads, it is routine practice to use six standard positions over the heart, starting on the right sternal border and following the general outline of the heart around to the left sternal border and then laterally as far as the midaxillary line.

To rule out the possibility of angina pectoris in an apparently normal subject who complains of precordial pain on exertion, Masters devised a scheme of controlled exercise to show abnormality in the electrocardiogram. After a routine tracing is taken, the patient ascends and descends a special two-step platform the number of times recommended for a person of his age and weight. Tracings of leads II and V_4 (at the cardiac apex) are made at stipulated intervals to demonstrate the effect of exercise and recovery to the resting state. Some changes in electric conductance are seen only in the

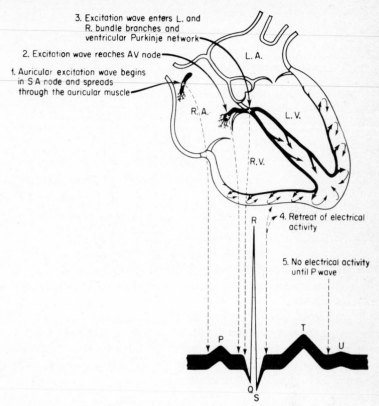

3. Excitation wave enters L. and
R. bundle branches and
ventricular Purkinje network

2. Excitation wave reaches AV node

1. Auricular excitation wave begins
in S A node and spreads
through the auricular muscle

L. A.

R. A.

L. V.

R. V.

R   4. Retreat of electrical
activity

5. No electrical activity
until P wave

T

P   U

Q
S

FIG. 10-1 The normal electrocardiogram. *(After Opal Hepler, "Manual of Clinical Laboratory Methods," 4th ed., 1954, by permission of Charles C Thomas, Publisher, Springfield, Ill.)*

tracings made immediately after, or shortly after, exercise. This test is called the Masters two-step.

A frequent, almost invariable, remark patients make when the technologist places the electrodes on his arms and legs is "This is just like the electric chair." Of course, nothing could be further from the truth. The flow of electric current, in minute intensities, is *from* the patient. He therefore feels nothing whatever during the course of the test.

Vectorcardiograms involve analysis of the electrocardiogram in order to determine the direction and strength of the impulses. These are obtained by a mathematical analysis.

ELECTROENCEPHALOGRAM

By an elaborate and delicate machine, electric impulses discharged by the brain cells are recorded on special paper for interpretation of possible abnormalities in the central nervous system. The electrodes of the electroencephalogram (EEG) machine are placed at specified points on the surface of the head and attached to the skin by an adhesive material. Because it involves the placement of electrodes on the head, the patient may be quite apprehensive about having the test done. The nurse can assure the patient there is no pain involved and that she will feel absolutely nothing, since the electrodes are picking up electric impulses of minute intensity that are discharged by her own brain cells. When the brain has been damaged or when the patient has epilepsy, the waves produced by the electric discharges are in patterns characteristic of the disease. Tracings are taken when the patient is awake, in hyperventilation (which may precipitate changes characteristic of grand mal seizures), and asleep.

An EEG usually takes about 2 h to complete. Careful pretest preparation is essential to the accuracy of the test. The neurologist who reads the tracings may give specific instructions, but, in general, the following preparation is basic:

1. On the day of the test, the patient takes no coffee, tea, Coca-Cola, or other such stimulant. Neither does she take alcohol (Alcohol is a depressant, of course, and would have a definite effect on the EEG).
2. On the day of the test, no medication is taken, except by special order of the physician.
3. The hair and scalp are thoroughly shampooed to remove all hair dressings and natural oils. After shampooing, no hair preparations of any sort may be used until after the tracing is completed.
4. Since a portion of the tracing is made with the patient asleep, it is helpful if the patient does not nap on the day of the test.

EXAMINATION OF BODY FLUIDS

Transudates

Transudates are fluids that accumulate in the body cavities, such as the pleural space, peritoneal space, and pericardial space, as the result of impaired circulation, which leads to passive congestion and edema. These fluids are not the result of an inflammatory process, and they differ from those that are. Transudates are clear, serous, and light-yellow in appearance. The specific gravity of such fluid is less than 1.018, and no clot forms. The protein content is low. Since it is noninflammatory, the fluid does not contain appreciable numbers of white blood cells, and bacteria are not found. When the fluid is part of a malignant process, the malignant cells may sometimes be found in the sediment.

Laboratory studies of transudates include inspection for appearance, testing for specific gravity, cell count, and protein determinations. Papanicolaou smears may be made of the sediment when a malignant condition is suspected.

Exudates

Exudates, the products of inflammatory processes, may collect in the body cavities as well as in the tissues. In contrast with transudates, exudates are characterized by a specific gravity higher than 1.018 and by a relatively high protein content. Although it may be clear in some cases, an exudate is usually cloudy due to the presence of white blood cells, red blood cells, etc., or chylous material. Frequently bacteria are found. Exudate fluid will clot spontaneously.

Laboratory studies of exudates include inspection for appearance, testing for specific gravity, cell counts, and protein determinations as well as smears and cultures for bacteria.

Synovial Fluid

Synovial fluid may be obtained by aspiration from a joint, bursa, or tendon sheath. Cell counts and smears and culture for bacteria are the usual tests done on synovial fluid in order to help determine the cause of increased fluid volume. It is normally clear and serous in appearance.

EXAMINATION OF STOOLS

General Considerations

As indicated in Chap. 8, microbiologic examinations of stool specimens are made to identify specific viruses, bacteria, fungi, or animal parasites that may be present in the intestinal tract. Other examinations may be done for occult blood and some chemical compounds.

Collection of Specimens for Culture

For virus cultures, stools must be treated immediately. If there is delay in the time between collection and starting the culture, the specimen must be kept cold. When the specimen is sent to another laboratory, it must be frozen and kept in dry ice for the transit period.

For bacterial cultures, stools must be examined immediately. Only a small amount of feces is necessary. With diarrheal stools, a large cotton swab dipped in the specimen, particularly the purulent-appearing patches, is quite satisfactory for culture. The swab is then placed in a sterile test tube for delivery to the laboratory. In bacillary dysentery, rectal swabs are a simple and satisfactory means of obtaining material. The anus is kept open with a tube, through which a large cotton swab is inserted to obtain material from the rectum. The swab is then placed in a sterile test tube for delivery to the laboratory.

Collection of Specimens for Parasites

Loose, fluid stools are likely to contain trophozoites of the intestinal amoebas and flagellates. These stools must be kept at body temperature and examined within 30 min of collection if the organisms are to be found in the active stage.

Well-formed or semiformed stools contain ova or the cystic forms of parasites, neither of which require maintenance of body temperature. They do not need to be kept warm or examined as quickly as fluid stools.

Collection of stools after purgative medication is an important step. The treatment for tapeworms is not complete unless the scolex (head) of the parasite is discharged from the intestine. Consequently, after medication to dislodge the scolex, a purgative is given, and *all the stools* in their entirety must be examined for the scolex.

Collection of Specimens for Occult Blood

A small amount of stool is all that is required for this examination. It need not be kept warm or examined immediately. If there is any doubt about the presence of a positive result, the patient should be on a meat-free diet for 3 days before the specimen is collected, since false positive results may occur from meat residue.

Collection of Specimens for Chemical Analysis

Since the amounts of the substances tested for are reported and calculated on the basis of daily output, the entire specimen should be sent to the laboratory. It is well to keep the specimen cold if there is to be a delay between collection and examination.

CHROMOSOME ANALYSIS

General Considerations

In keeping with and aiding the development of the understanding of disease on the molecular level, chromosome analysis has assumed a very important place in diagnostic procedures. In order to understand the principles involved in this procedure, a brief review of the development of our knowledge of chromosomes is necessary.

Gregor Mendel, in 1865, reported his experiments on common

garden peas, which laid the foundation for the basic laws of heredity. It was not until 1900, however, that the significance of his findings and theories was recognized and further work done to elaborate on his foundation. It is now common knowledge that chromosomes are the messengers of heredity through the millions of genes of which they are made and that deoxyribonucleic acid (DNA) is the basic genetic material. The arrangement of the base pairs within the DNA molecule constitutes the genetic codes which determine the characteristics of the individual, as well as those of the general species to which the individual belongs. Species breed true because DNA duplicates an exact copy of itself as cells grow and divide. The genetic code is subject to injury and alteration, and these vulnerabilities result in functional as well as structural defects. An example of a functional defect is PKU, which is due to an absence of an enzyme. Cleft palate is an example of a genetically determined structural defect.

Meiosis and Mitosis

The nucleus of every cell in the individual has the same number of chromosomes, the number being species specific. In man, there are 46 chromosomes, including 44 autosomes and 2 sex chromosomes. The autosomes occur in pairs, one unit of the pair from each parent. The sex chromosomes, X for female and Y for male, occur in combination as well, with genotypes being XX for female and XY for male.

MEIOSIS

The germ cells, spermatozoa and ova, are the only cells of the body which do not have 46 chromosomes. In the generation of these cells, the chromosomes are halved, so that each mature germ cell normally has one of each kind of chromosome; the total is 23, the haploid number. This process of reduction in the phenomenon of replication of germ cells is termed meiosis. Abnormalities in meiosis, termed "nondisjunction," can result in germ cells that have more or less than 23 chromosomes. Should conception then occur and the offspring live, he will fail to have the normal number of chromosomes. An example is Down's syndrome (mongolism), in which the individual has 47 chromosomes.

MITOSIS

In all the other cell replications, the chromosomes within the nucleus grow and divide in the process of "mitosis," a splitting of the nucleus into two identical cells with the full complement of chromosomes in each. There are five stages, or phases, in mitosis: interphase, prophase, metaphase, anaphase, and telophase. At interphase, the usual metabolic processes of the cell are going on. Prophase is the beginning stage of replication, with the initial changes in the nucleus. Proceeding to metaphase, the chromosomes are aligned singly in an equatorial fashion around the nucleus. During anaphase, the chromosomes split, with each half migrating to one of the two poles of the cell. During telephase, the cell wall divides, and two distinct and complete daughter cells result; each of them enters interphase, beginning the entire process again.

Methods of Chromosome Analysis

With the advent of tissue cultures, a practical method of studying chromosomes in man and animals was developed. The cells used for this purpose may be leukocytes (from peripheral blood), bone marrow, or skin. Most commonly, the leukocytes are used. The cells are grown in vitro. After the appropriate time to allow the growing cells to reach metaphase, the culture is treated chemically to prevent further mitosis. The cells are then treated to break the membranes, releasing the chromosomes intact. After staining, photomicrographs are made of the sample. From prints of the photomicrographs, the chromosomes are separated, then matched according to size and morphology. The autosomes are labeled numerically in descending order according to size. The resulting pattern is called a *karyotype;* Fig. 10-2 illustrates the normal female karyotype. By studying the number and morphology of the chromosomes, certain diagnoses may be made. For example, sporadic mongolism is the result of an abnormality in chromosome 21, with three, rather than the normal

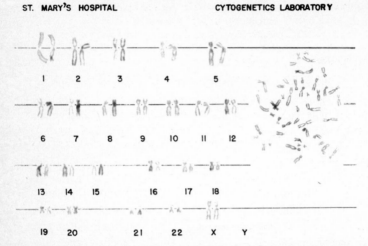

FIG. 10-2 Normal female karyotype showing matched pairs of autosomal chromosomes (1 to 22) and sex chromosomes (X). Inset: photomicrograph from which the typing is made. *(Cytogenetics Laboratory, St. Mary's Hospital, St. Louis, Mo.)*

two, of these chromosomes being present. This is an example of trisomy. The presence of extra chromosomes, although resulting in abnormalities, is apparently not lethal; whereas the absence of an autosome is lethal.

Use of Chromosome Analysis

While knowledge of the characteristics controlled by each chromosome is still limited, enough is known to make this area of study helpful in certain diagnoses and a fertile field for future application. Chromosome analysis provides valuable information in a number of conditions, such as the following:

1. Distinguishing cretinism from mongolism
2. Intersex problems
3. Infertility problems
4. Primary amenorrhea

TABLE 10-1 RELATIONSHIP BETWEEN SEX CHROMOSOMES
AND FUNCTION

Condition	Sex chromosomes present	Phenotype	Characteristics
Normal male	XY	Male	Normal
Normal female	XX	Female	Normal
Turner's syndrome	XO	Female	Infertility, physical abnormalities
Klinefelter's syndrome	XXY	Male	Eunuchoid, infertility
X trisomy	XXX	Female	Mental retardation, infertility

5. Certain types of mental retardation
6. Multiple congenital abnormalities

SEMINAL-FLUID ANALYSIS

Examination of semen is one of the procedures used in evaluation of the barren marriage. Sperm counts are also used to monitor effectiveness of sterilization by severing the vas deferens in men wishing this operation. The specimen is usually obtained by masturbation, although the patient may prefer one of the other methods because of religious or aesthetic reasons. These methods are associated with coitus. In coitus interruptus, normal intercourse is pursued, but the penis is withdrawn from the vagina just prior to ejaculation, and the semen is collected in a clean glass jar. If a condom is used, the full cycle of coitus may be completed, since the semen is collected in the condom. After collection, the condom is tied and placed in a clean jar. Catholic patients may use a plastic sheath[1] with a small perforation and collect the specimen during normal coitus.

Several precautions must be observed for accurate results. No matter where (at home or in the physician's office) the specimen is collected, it should be delivered to the laboratory in no less than

[1] Milex Seminal Pouch, Milex Products, Chicago, Ill.

2 h, and chilling must be avoided. If a condom or sheath is used, it must be washed with soap and water, rinsed thoroughly, and completely dried before use. A 3-day period of continence before collection of the specimen is usually recommended.

Semen first coagulates (within about 20 min) and then liquifies spontaneously (in an additional 30 min) into a transluscent, turbid, viscid fluid. Table 10-2 summarizes normal results.

AMNIOTIC-FLUID ANALYSIS

In addition to the usefulness of analysis of amniotic fluid in relation to the status of the fetus subject to hemolytic disease of the newborn, this area of investigation is growing as a means of early identification of genetic abnormalities. Prenatal diagnosis involves a team: the genetic counselor, obstetrician, pediatrician, and laboratory cytogeneticist. Amniocentesis and the subsequent study of the fluid and cells is not an entity of itself but part of the approach to prenatal diagnosis. Undoubtedly, liberalization of abortion restrictions has raised the possibility of terminating pregnancies in which the fetus is likely to have a genetic abnormality that would seriously compromise life or function. Moral and ethical dilemmas are inextricably bound to the onus upon each team member, including the patient, calling for the utmost care in decision-making.

TABLE 10-2   ANALYSIS OF NORMAL SEMINAL FLUID

Characteristic	Normal value
Liquification	Within 30 min
Morphology	More than 70% normal mature spermatozoa
Motility	More than 60% of spermatozoa actively mobile
pH	7.0–8.0
Count	60–150 million/ml
Volume	1.5–5.0 ml

SOURCE: From Israel Davidsohn and John B. Henry (eds.), "Todd-Sanford Clinical Diagnosis by Laboratory Methods," W. B. Saunders Company, Philadelphia, 1969.

The translation of genetics research into clinical practice, even on a limited basis, has led to oversimplification and, in some instances, assumptions that amniocentesis and amniotic-fluid analysis for genetic studies are no more complicated than a blood test and that they offer most of the answers to complex questions. By no means is this the case. Amniocentesis is an aid to the diagnosis of only a few abnormalities. In addition, it is not always possible to obtain results early enough in pregnancy to allow therapeutic abortion. Finally, the procedures require specially equipped and staffed laboratories. Unwarranted expectations are among the problems with which the team must deal, underlining the importance of the qualified genetic counselor in particular.

The basic decision of whether to proceed with amniocentesis must be made on an individual basis, considering the possibilities and the seriousness of a genetic problem. In essence, it is a matter of determining as accurately as possible what the alternative risks may be. Time is also a critical element. There is approximately 80 percent success in culturing the cells from amniotic fluid. Amniocentesis cannot be done before 14- to 20-weeks gestation, culture of cells and biochemical studies require from 4 to 6 weeks to complete. The question then arises as to whether the information obtained will be available within the limits for a therapeutic abortion, should that be the decision.

Even though many genetically related diseases are well-defined, there are those, such as sicklemia and the classic hemophilias, which cannot be diagnosed in utero. Diagnosis of these diseases depends upon body constituents inaccessible prenatally. There are some diagnostic tests on the amniotic fluid itself that yield information on some of the inborn errors of metabolism. Many of the procedures require cultured cells for karyotyping or biochemical tests for enzymes known to be the basis of inborn errors of metabolism. Table 10-3 shows the procedures related to conditions that may be in utero. As with practically all diagnostic problems, the combination of clinical findings and history with the information generated by the laboratory is essential.[1]

[1] A clear explanation of the complexities, advantages and disadvantages of amniocentesis and amniotic-fluid analysis is given by Dr. Lawrence Karp in Amniocentesis Is Not Just a Laboratory Test, *Med. Dimensions,* 3(5):23–26 May, 1974.

TABLE 10-3   AMNIOTIC-FLUID ANALYSIS IN GENETIC DIAGNOSIS

Condition	Karo-type*	Biochemical Tests*	Fluid Analysis
Chromosomal disorders			
Trisomy 21 (Down's syndrome), trisomy D, trisomy E, sex-chromosome aneuploidies, translocations, structural abberrations	✓		
Sex-linked-recessive disorders			
Fabry's disease, Lesch-Nyhan syndrome		Enzymes	
Hunter's syndrome		^{35}S uptake	Dermatan sulfate, heparitin sulfate
Autosomal-recessive disorders			
Lipid metabolism: Tay-Sach's disease, Niemann-Pick disease, metachromatic leukodystrophy, Gaucher's disease, GM$_1$ ganglio-siderosis, Krabbe's disease		Enzymes	
Mucopolysaccharidoses: Hurler's syndrome		^{35}S uptake	Dermatan sulfate, heparitin sulfate
Amino acid disorders			
Maple syrup urine disease		Enzyme	
Methylmalonic aciduria			Methylmal-onic acid
Cystinosis		Elevated nonprotein cystine	
Carbohydrate-metabolism disorders			
Glycogen storage, type II; galactosemia		Enzymes	
Miscellaneous diseases			
Lysosomal acid phosphatase deficiency		Enzyme	
Androgenital syndrome			17-Keto-steroid†
Multifactoral disorders			
Anecephaly, spina bifida, meningomye-locele			α-Feto-protein

*Requires cell culture.   †In third trimester only.

SOURCE: Adapted from Lawrence Kark, Amniocentesis Is Not Just a Labora-tory test, *Med. Dimensions*, 3(5):23–26, May, 1974.

REFERENCES

Davidsohn, Israel, and John B. Henry (eds.): "Todd-Sanford Clinical Diagnosis by Laboratory Methods," 15th ed., Saunders, Philadelphia, 1974.

Diamond, E. Grey: "Electrocardiography," Williams & Wilkins, Baltimore, 1955.

Freeman, J. A., and M. F. Beeler: "Laboratory Medicine—Clinical Microscopy," Lea & Febiger, Philadelphia, 1974.

Hampton, Clarita: Understanding Chromosome Analysis, *Amer. J. Med. Techn.,* **30**(5):321, 1964.

Kark, Lawrence: Amniocentesis Is Not Just a Laboratory Test, *Med. Dimensions,* 3(5):23–26, May, 1974.

Nadler, H. L., and A. B. Gerbie: Role of Amniocentesis in the Intrauterine Detection of Genetic Disorders, *New Eng. J. Med.,* **282**:596, 1970.

Nora, James J., and F. Clarke Fraser: "Medical Genetics: Principles and Practice," Lea & Febiger, Philadelphia, 1974.

Priest, Jean: "Cytogenetics," Lea & Febiger, Philadelphia, 1969.

ELEVEN

RADIOLOGIC EXAMINATIONS

HISTORY AND DEVELOPMENT OF X-RAY

Discovered in 1895 by Wilhelm Konrad Röntgen, the phenomenon of x-radiation was greeted by the medical profession with unbounded enthusiasm as a valuable, almost miraculous, aid to diagnosis and treatment of disease. Many machines were installed, and many different diseases were treated by workers who knew little or nothing of the potent force with which they were dealing. Indeed, even those most learned in the field were unaware of the consequences of the kind of energy they were applying. Only after the deleterious effects of uncontrolled x-radiation and its failure to cure various diseases as hoped became apparent, was a concerted effort begun to standardize and control x-radiation and to protect both patient and operator. By 1906, use of x-radiation had fallen somewhat into disrepute, but by 1910 the machines and methods of control had been improved, and the field began its second phase, gaining in stature and usefulness by continuing efforts to harness this powerful adjunct to medicine's arsenal of weapons against disease. An eminent physician once stated that "apart from bacteriology, which, like medicine is biological in approach, no discovery in pure science has been of such signal service to the practice of medicine and surgery as that of x-rays."

Present-day radiology has gained the confidence of both the physician and the public, and the value and limitations of this field have been established. Scientific and public concern for greater protection against harmful effects have, over the past few years, elicited even greater efforts toward even more precise handling of irradiation equipment. This is the pattern of development of radiology: the period of unlimited enthusiasm that proverbially greets a major discovery; the period of relative disillusionment and disappointment; the period of growth toward maturity through increased knowledge; and now a period of refinement in precision of judgment and equipment.

As is the case with all scientific discoveries, the actual unlocking of the door in a given area of investigation depends upon the work of many minds, and the person who is given the honor of unlocking it is actually using his predecessors' findings and putting them together in proper sequence. Thus, the happy accident does not just happen, it results from the right combination of facts, observations, and induction on the part of a prepared mind. Such was the case with Röntgen, the German physicist whose name is forever attached to the field of radiology. While repeating some experiments of other workers in the field, he had the right combination to unlock the door to x-radiation. The discovery of x-rays on November 8, 1895 by Röntgen was the result of systematic investigation. It is said that he himself remarked when he first noticed the effects of x-rays, "I did not think. I investigated."

NOMENCLATURE

Since he did not know the exact origin or mechanism of the rays he discovered, Röntgen called them x-rays, borrowing the symbol for the unknown from algebraic equations. Although a great deal is now known about these rays, they are still called by their discoverer's original name; sometimes they are called roentgen rays. The nomenclature of this area of study is derived from combinations of terms that describe properties of x-rays and the uses to which they are put. For example, the study of this specialty is roentgenology. The broader term, radiology, is also used synonymously, although it includes the study and use of radioactive elements as well. The medical specialist, therefore, is a *roentgenologist* or *radiologist*. The films that comprise the tools of diagnosis are referred to as *roentgenograms* or *radiographs*. The two suffixes *gram* and *graph* are derived from the Greek words "gamma," and "graphein," meaning "written" or "drawn." Films of specific areas of the body may have specific names, e.g., cholecystogram for gallbladder visualization.

MEASUREMENT OF X-RADIATION

The unit of measurement of x-ray and gamma-ray intensity is the *roentgen* (r). The roentgen has been standardized as the quantity of x- or gamma radiation that will produce an electrical change of one electrostatic unit on 0.00193 g air. Although the roentgen was originally developed for use as a unit of radiologic dose, workers in physics and radiobiology also use the roentgen and a number of units derived from it. Ordinary exposure to this type of radiation is of small magnitude, and in order to express this, the term *milliroentgen* (mr) is used. This is 1/1000 of a roentgen.

TYPES OF RADIOLOGIC EXAMINATION

There are three methods of examination with use of x-rays: taking "pictures" by exposure of the part to x-rays with film to record the results; exposing the part to x-rays and visualizing the results by use of the fluoroscopic screen; and a combination of these two methods, which records the results on photographic film in miniature. In tomography (also called planigraphy), a procedure of successive exposures at calculated depths is used in order to localize otherwise obscured structures. It is used with caution, since it increases the amount of radiation exposure.

Radiographs

A radiograph, or x-ray "picture," is made using special film for the purpose, the film is held in a cassette (Fig. 11-1). Unlike photographic film, x-ray film has emulsion, the carrier for the light-sensitive chemicals, on both sides of the cellulose acetate base. The device used to hold the film, the cassette, is a light-proof case of special construction, which incorporates intensifying screens of calcium tungstate on a sheet of cardboard backing. These screens intensify, or increase, the photographic effect of the x-rays, since the calcium tungstate crystals glow, or fluoresce, when struck by the x-rays. By this aid, much clearer and sharper images are produced on the x-ray film without extra exposure of the patient to x-radiation.

X-ray film is processed in much the same manner as photographic film. Developing reduces the silver halide to metallic silver in direct proportion to the amount of exposure of the material

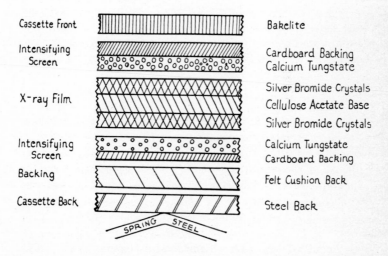

Cassette Front	Bakelite
Intensifying Screen	Cardboard Backing / Calcium Tungstate
X-ray Film	Silver Bromide Crystals / Cellulose Acetate Base / Silver Bromide Crystals
Intensifying Screen	Calcium Tungstate / Cardboard Backing
Backing	Felt Cushion Back
Cassette Back	Steel Back

SPRING STEEL

FIG. 11-1 Cross section of a cassette. *(From Isadore Meschan, "Roentgen Signs in Clinical Diagnosis," W. B. Saunders Company, Philadelphia, 1956, by permission of the author and publisher.)*

TABLE 11-1   RADIOLUCENCY AND RADIOPACITY OF TISSUES AND
OTHER MEDICALLY IMPORTANT SUBSTANCES

Very radiolucent	Moderately radiolucent	Intermediate	Moderately radiopaque	Very radiopaque
Gas	Fatty tissue	Connective tissues	Bone	Heavy metals
		Muscle tissue	Calcium salts	
		Blood		
		Cartilage		
		Epithelium		
		Cholesterol stones		
		Uric acid stones		

SOURCE: From Isadore Meschan, "Atlas of Normal Radiographic Anatomy,"
2d ed., W. B. Saunders Company, Philadelphia, 1959, by permission of the
publisher.

during the radiologic procedure, thus bringing out the image. A
second processing solution—the fixer, or hypo—completes the
film preparation. This solution dissolves away the unexposed silver
halide, hardens the gelatin in the emulsion on the film, and preserves
the film from discoloration. After proper development and fixation,
the film is washed well and dried.

Fluroscopic Examination

This procedure is derived from the phenomenon of fluorescence,
which some chemical compounds demonstrate. This was referred to
above in the discussion of intensifying screens. In this type of x-ray
examination, the patient is placed in front of an x-ray tube, and the
mobile fluoroscopic screen is held over the part to be examined. The
screen is composed of calcium tungstate crystals, which fluoresce
when struck by x-rays, thus casting an image, or shadow, on the
screen. The less dense parts of the body allow more x-rays to pass,
thus producing light areas on the screen; conversely, the denser
parts prohibit passage of x-rays, resulting in dark areas on the screen.
Since the contrast between light and dark areas is quite delicate, the

procedure must be carried out in the dark. This requires the radio-logist to accommodate his eyes to darkness in order that he see well and is not tempted to overexpose the patient to get sharp definition of images on the fluorographic screen.

Most fluoroscopic units now have an attachment that makes it possible for the radiologist to expose films of areas that he particularly wants to study at leisure and that he would be unable to obtain with the usual radiographs. These are known as spot films and are a valuable aid to diagnosis, and they reduce the time required for ade-quate fluoroscopic examination. A television attachment with image intensifier is also available.

Photofluorograms

In this procedure, the image is cast upon a built-in fluoroscopic screen; simultaneously, a small photograph is taken on photographic film. The film is usually 70 mm square per exposure. Photofluoro-grams are precise enough to detect possible abnormality but not sufficiently so to be conclusively diagnostic. Any suspicious or ques-tionable film taken in this fashion must be followed by a regular radiograph in order to confirm or rule out abnormality.

This procedure is, by nature and intent, a screening process. It is a great deal less expensive in time, materials, and labor than regular x-ray examinations of the chest. There is convenience to the patient because complete disrobing is not required. The small film can be easily incorporated with the patient's record if desired.

Cineradiography

As the name indicates, this form of radiography provides a motion-picture record of an examination. By a special attachment to the fluoroscopic apparatus, photographic film is exposed in a manner similar to that of the motion-picture camera, although the number of frames exposed is fewer, and the time interval between frames is slightly longer. Through the use of cineradiography, the radiologist is able to study the events he has seen on fluoroscopy, some of which may have been so fleeting that is impossible to make sound judgments. In addition, the influence of motion is important to the diagnosis of certain conditions. This technique is particularly valuable in diagnosis of pathology in the urinary tract, especially the urethra. With cineradiography, there is opportunity to study the flow of fluid (containing a radiopaque substance) from the bladder as the patient voids, thus outlining the urethra. Prior to this, diagnosis of urethral strictures was quite difficult, which led to a misdiagnosis of hydroureter when it was assumed that the abnormality causing this condition was higher up in the urinary system.

POSITIONING THE PATIENT

Obviously, the position of the patient when a film is made will affect the appearance of the radiograph. It is essential to interpretation of the radiographic findings to know the patient's position in order to localize the lesions or foreign bodies that are visualized. For this reason, the various positions are indicated in the reports of

TABLE 11-2   PATIENT POSITIONS FOR RADIOGRAPHY

Position	Abbreviation	Definition
Posteroanterior	PA	Front of body next to film holder; x-ray beam passes from back to front of body
Anteroposterior	AP	Back of body next to film holder; x-ray beam passes from front to back of body
Lateral	Rt. lat.	Right side next to film holder
	Lt. lat.	Left side next to film holder
Oblique	Obl. (rt. or	Obl. ant.: body at an angle, with the front
Anterior	lt.) ant.	side closest to film holder
Posterior	or post.	Obl. post.: body at an angle, with the back side of body closest to film holder
Decubitus	Rt. lat.	Patient lies on his side; the film is in front
	Lt. lat.	or in back of him, as indicated by AP or PA
Erect		Patient stands or sits upright when film is taken
Semierect		Patient lies at a 45° angle to the beam of x-rays

the radiologist (see Table 11-2). A basic working principle in positioning is that the part to be studied should be next to the film. Thus, in studies of the spinal column, the patient lies on his back with the film beneath him. In describing the position of the patient, the terms refer first to the x-ray beam and then to the x-ray exit surface.

CONTRAST MEDIA

Contrast media include materials that alter radiopacity of one part in comparison with the surrounding parts. Contrast media are essential to the visualization of certain body cavities. The contrast media are introduced to the desired area by several means. In gastrointestinal studies, the patient drinks a suspension of barium sulfate for studies of the upper portion of the gastrointestinal tract and is given an enema of a suspension of barium sulfate for studies of the colon. Radiopaque dyes that are concentrated by the gallbladder are

TABLE 11-3   CONTRAST MEDIA

Medium	Region visualized
Gaseous: air, helium, oxygen, carbon dioxide	Ventricles, meningeal spaces of the brain, subarachnoid spaces, pleural space, perirenal tissues, urinary bladder, colon (after evacuation of barium enema), stomach (with barium for double contrast)
Insoluble salts of heavy metals: barium sulfate, bismuth carbonate	Gastrointestinal tract
Organic insoluble iodides: Priodax, Telepaque, Teridax	Gallbladder
Organic soluble iodides: Diodrast, Neo-iopaz, Cholografin, Urokon	Urinary tract, heart and great vessels, peripheral vessels, gallbladder (direct, at surgery), bronchial tree, fistulous tracts, paranasal sinuses, salivary ducts, seminal vesicles, urethra, uterus, fallopian tubes, subarachnoid spaces
Colloidal suspensions: Skiodan acacia, Salpix	Uterus and fallopian tubes

given by mouth the evening before the examination is to be made. In pyelograms, the radiopaque dye may be given intravenously and concentrated in the kidneys by the mechanism of excretion, or it may be introduced into the renal pelvises and urinary system by the retrograde manner at cystoscopy.

THERAPEUTIC USES OF X-RAYS

Superficial Treatment

In superficial therapeutic use of x-rays, various skin disorders are treated, e.g., severe acne and plantar warts. In these treatments, the "soft" (gamma) rays are used because penetration is not necessary. As with all treatment procedures, the radiologist determines dosage and supervises the x-ray technician in administering the treatment.

Deep Treatment

Deep therapeutic use of x-rays is utilized in the treatment of malignant conditions and certain leukemias and for intentional sterilization. The "hard" (beta) waves are necessary in this procedure because they penetrate well and are more effective in cell destruction. The radiologist determines dosage, positions the patient, and sets the direction of the x-ray beam.

NECESSARY PRECAUTIONS IN USING X-RAYS

General Considerations

It has long been known that too much exposure to x-radiation produces deleterious effects. These may be brought about either by repeated exposure to relatively low intensities over a long period of time or by single exposures to high intensities. The low intensities are referred to as "soft" radiation and are used in diagnostic and superficial therapeutic procedures. The soft radiation utilizes the relatively long waves of the x-ray spectrum, which do not penetrate deeply, as do the relatively short waves. The short x-ray waves are utilized in deep treatment. When the soft waves strike an object, they tend to break down into shorter waves, resulting in the phenomenon known as secondary radiation. It is secondary radiation that is the most damaging. In order to prevent secondary radiation in x-ray examinations, aluminum filters and lead protective devices are used to absorb it.

The Atomic Energy Commission has established the maximum permissable dose to persons working with radiation at 300 mr/week of whole body radiation. Devices for measuring the cumulative dosage of radiation received have been developed and are worn by technicians in order that accurate measurements of exposure can be made. The National Academy of Science estimates that the average American receives 3 r/year from all diagnostic x-rays. In the first 30 years of his life, if he had one 14 x 17 chest film each year, the gonadal dose would amount of 0.05 r. The total upper limit for such dosage has been set at 10 r. Thus, reasonable safety is possible.

In considering exposure to x-radiation, it is well to remember the importance of the body surface area that is exposed. For comparison, consider burns: A light burn over a wide area is more serious than an intense burn in a small area. This is true of x-radiation exposure too. For the usual diagnostic use of x-rays, the exposure is limited in time, intensity, and body area as much as possible. It has been shown that 400- to 600-r exposure of the whole body once kills half the animals so exposed in 30 days. By contrast, therapeutic doses of 4,000 to 5,000 r to a limited area are compatible with life, causing destruction of a limited number and area of cells in the body.

Dr. William J. Tuddenham, Assistant Professor of Radiology at the Hospital of the University of Pennsylvania, has said that although the ultimate responsibility for controlling the hazard of medical x-ray exposure lies with the radiologist, it is one that must be shared by many others. He points out that

    . . . it is in part the responsibility of the referring doctor who can best assess the clinical indications for study, and who, by pertinent information, can guide the radiologist. It is in part the responsibility of the patient, who, by following directions carefully, can ensure proper preparation and thus obviate the need for repeat examinations, and who, by providing an accurate history, can also guide the radiologist and reduce the exposure needed to reach a diagnosis. It is in part the responsibility of the hospital administration which is often responsible for providing the radiologist with safe, modern equipment.

Dr. Tuddenham further remarks, "What is rarely understood by the public, however, is that diagnostic x-ray exposures, as currently used on the average individual by reputable doctors are nowhere near the upper limits of safety that have been set, and that most fears are thus not justified."[1] The radiologist must weigh the risks involved to the patient's health and life.

Questions that commonly arise in the lay person's mind in regard to exposure to x-rays as they affect the gonads are whether it leads to sterility, loss of libido, and loss of vigor; whether reproductive organs become radioactive of themselves; whether overexposure will result in monster children. None of these events occur. Sterility may be induced by special treatment of the gonadal area, but this does not happen in ordinary diagnostic procedures.

Deleterious Effects of X-rays

Maximal exposure within safe limits so far as superficial injuries are concerned is 1 r/day. This is confined to a small area and does not expose the whole body.

SUPERFICIAL INJURY

The following injuries are produced by prolonged "light" exposure

1. Burn simulating severe sunburn (immediate reaction)
2. Thin, scaly skin
3. Telangiectasis

[1] Hospitals Can Keep Patients from Developing Nuclear Neurosis, *Mod. Hosp.*, 93(3):90, 1959.

4. Striation and brittle nails
5. Keratoses
6. Carcinoma

INJURY TO HEMATOPOIETIC TISSUES

Anemia, leukemia, and leukopenia have been shown to occur more frequently in persons repeatedly exposed to radiation, such as radiologists and technicians. In man, the maximum permissible dose is not known as far as the hematopoietic system is concerned. As would be expected, this cannot be determined by experimentation.

CARCINOGENESIS

It has long been known that frequent low-grade exposure to radiation can result in highly malignant skin lesion. For this reason, workers in the field must protect themselves carefully; e.g., the doctor who performs fluoroscopic examinations must wear lead-lined gloves and apron and avoid exposing unprotected areas of the body to the x-ray beam.

Protection of Patients and Personnel

Since exposure techniques and calculations of dosage are highly technical, no attempt will be made here to outline these factors. The major considerations are to use maximum filtration of the primary beam, to use higher voltages in order to penetrate the skin and reduce the necessary exposure time, to narrow the field of radiation, and to hold fluoroscopic examinations to as short a time as possible.

Technicians who must, by the nature of their work, be repeatedly exposed to radiation are sometimes forced to call upon nursing personnel to aid in holding patients for radiologic examinations. With the possible hazard uppermost in mind, the radiology department will not require nursing personnel to assist when it will endanger them, either by frequency of exposure or because of some individual susceptibility. Whenever the assistance of the nurse is necessary, he will be provided with a lead-rubber apron to protect him from radiation.

The patient who is to undergo radiologic examination frequently asks questions about the dangers of exposure to x-rays. She may even be adamant about not having radiographs taken. It is important, therefore, that the nurse understand the values and limitations of radiologic procedures and be able to assure her that all possible care is being taken to ensure her safety. When he is asked for specific information about how much exposure the patient is likely to receive, it is probably best to tell her to ask the x-ray technician or the radiologist, since they have the information and know what films will be necessary for her particular examination.

PREPARATION OF PATIENTS FOR X-RAY EXAMINATIONS

It is recognized that individual radiology departments have their own particular methods and required nursing procedures for preparing and transporting patients to the department for examination. The following instructions are considered standard and indicate the rationale involved in each procedure.

Intravenous Pyelogram

Since fecal matter and gas in the intestinal tract obscure the urinary-tract structures, it is necessary to clear as much of this from the lower bowel as possible. This is done by a combination of castor oil and enemas. The evening meal should be light (tea, toast, fruit), and no food or fluids are allowed after 9 P.M. the evening prior to examination or in the morning until the examination is completed. At the time of examination, contrast medium that will be excreted by the kidneys is given intravenously. Films are made at given time intervals to observe the rate of excretion, the concentration of the contrast medium in the kidney calices and pelvises, and the outline of the ureters and urinary bladder. Retrograde pyelography is used when the contrast-medium-excretion procedure is inadequate or when special studies of renal anatomy are indicated.

The patient may be told that at least two venipunctures will be done and that the examination will take about 1 h.

Cholecystogram

As with pyelography, clearing the intestinal tract of as much fecal material and gas as possible is necessary for adequate visualization of the gallbladder. This is accomplished by enemas and a mild cathartic, which is included in the tablets of dye (contrast medium) administered. The patient is given a light supper of tea and toast. No cream or butter may be used for this meal, since fats stimulate the gallbladder, which must be at rest in order to concentrate the dye well. The tablets of contrast medium are given to the patient after the evening meal. Usually the patient takes six tablets, allowing 5 min between each tablet. Nothing is allowed the patient by mouth until the examination is completed. The patient should be told to expect some diarrhea after taking the tablets and that he need not be concerned about it, since it is part of the procedure to clear the intestinal tract. After the films of the dye-filled gallbladder have been made, the patient is given a fatty meal to stimulate the gallbladder to empty, and a film is taken to judge this function. The time required for the examination is about 1 h, excluding the time allowed for the fatty-meal effect.

Cholangiogram

Cholangiography is a means of visualizing the cystic, hepatic, and common ducts. The intravenous technique is sometimes used, although the results are not as conclusive as those provided by other methods. In this technique, the dye is selectively excreted by the liver into the biliary tract. Films are made at intervals beginning at 10 min after injection of the dye and continuing until the height of concentration and the beginning flow into the intestinal tract. This usually takes about 4 h. In preparation for the procedure, the patient is dehydrated by restricting fluid intake, and the intestinal tract is cleared by castor oil and enemas.

The postoperative cholangiogram technique utilizes the drainage tube left in place at surgery on the gallbladder and associated structures. The dye is injected into the drain, and films are made immediately. Normally the biliary structures fill readily, and the dye enters the intestine without delay.

The operative cholangiogram technique affords the opportunity to inject the contrast medium into the common duct under direct vision during the exploratory operation on the biliary structures. The anesthetist suspends the patient's breathing momentarily with curarelike drugs, and a film is immediately obtained of the area. Such films aid the surgeon in localizing possible stones that would be missed by manual examination and reveal any stones higher in the biliary tree.

Barium Enema

Obviously, the colon must be cleared of fecal material before a successful examination by barium enema can be done. This is accomplished by giving the patient castor oil the day before examination, a liquid supper, and enemas at prescribed times. Nothing is allowed by mouth until the examination is completed. The time required for the examination itself is usually 15 to 30 min. The patient may be informed that he will have an enema consisting of a solution that will make his colon radiopaque and that he will have to hold the enema until the films are made.

At the time of the examination, the radiologist fluoroscopically observes the filling of the colon by the suspension of barium sulfate. When the fluoroscopic examination is completed, films are made of the filled colon and then the patient evacuates the contrast material. If indicated, double-contrast examination may be done. This is accomplished by filling the colon with air after evacuation of the barium sulfate. The mucosa of the colon retains a sufficient coating of barium so that, when air is injected, the radiolucent area of the air is outlined. By this means, polypoid masses are better visualized.

Gastrointestinal Tests

No special preparation for this examination is necessary, except that the patient is not allowed anything by mouth from the evening meal the night before until after the examination is completed. It is necessary that the stomach be empty in order to accommodate the barium meal and also to avoid complications in case the patient is nauseated. The radiologist observes the filling of the stomach as the patient drinks a suspension of barium sulfate. Some films are made immediately, some during, and others after the fluoroscopic examination. The time required for the examination is about 30 min. The patient may have his meals afterward, and a follow-up film is made 24 h after the barium meal. The patient should be informed that his stool will be very light in color after the examination because of the passage of the barium sulfate.

MISCELLANEOUS RADIOLOGIC EXAMINATIONS

The remaining radiographic examinations require special skill and technique and are done only under special circumstances, as indicated.

Pneumoencephalogram

This is a roentgenographic picture of the ventricles and meningeal spaces after introduction of air into the subarachnoid space. It is sometimes done to localize space-filling abnormalities of the brain and meninges. Headache is a common aftereffect.

Ventriculogram

This is a roentgenogram of the ventricles of the brain after the introduction of air. Headache is particularly an aftereffect of this examination. The patient should be instructed to lie flat for some time after the examination in order to minimize the headache.

Myelogram

This is a roentgenogram of the subarachnoid space of the spinal column. It may be accomplished by injection of air or one of the iodized compounds as contrast medium. If the latter is used, as much of it as possible is removed after completion of the examination.

Cardioangiogram

In this procedure, the heart and great vessels are visualized. An organic iodide medium is injected rapidly into the heart, and films are made in rapid succession in two planes to study the anatomy of the heart and great vessels. Catheterization of the heart is required.

Bronchogram

A bronchogram is a roentgenographic picture of the bronchial tree. One of the soluble iodides is instilled in the bronchi by an atomizer in order to visualize these structures. Films are made immediately after the instillation.

Hysterosalpingogram

This is a roentgenogram of the uterus and fallopian tubes. Contrast medium is injected through the cervical canal, and films are made to demonstrate the morphology and patency of the uterus and the tubes.

Mammography

A technique using special film and different factors for exposure has been developed which makes it possible to study the tissue of the breast radiographically. This technique is used in preliminary diagnosis of breast cancer and for differentiating malignant from nonmalignant nodules in the breast. While mammography will not be used as a substitute for biopsy, there are important uses which make it a valuable diagnostic tool. As mentioned above, differentiation in fibrocystic disease is possible. In large, fatty breasts, mammography is important because the presence of a nodule can be defined radiographically when the clinician can feel nothing. As a follow-up procedure in patients who have had a mastectomy, periodic examination of the remaining breast by mammography can help to detect early lesions which might appear. Early detection of lesions too small to produce symptoms is also possible. The interpretation and diagnosis of lesions by this method, is, of course, dependent to a significant degree on the skills of the x-ray technologist and the radiologist.

Dacryocystography

When the lacrimal passage is inadequate or obstructed, normal secretion of tears cannot be accommodated. The dacryocystogram is useful in locating the site and nature of obstructive epiphora. A contrast medium is introduced into the passageway to outline the structure. Since local anesthetic is used, the patient must be cautioned to avoid dust or other particulate matter until feeling is restored. The procedure is contraindicated in the presence of infection.

Sialography

Visualization of the parotid or submandibular glands is used to demonstrate the structure of the ducts and possible stones. After films are made and assessed for technical quality, the patient is given lemon or an acid drop to suck in order to stimulate emptying of the contrast medium from the gland.

Pneumoperitoneum Radiography

Air, oxygen, carbon dioxide, or nitrous oxide gas may be injected into the abdomen to assist in visualization of the diaphragm, the exterior stomach wall, or the pelvic viscera. The amount of gas introduced and the positioning of the patient are major factors in the success of the procedure. The large bowel must be cleared of fecal material and gas for optimal visualization of structures.

Pneumomediastinography

This procedure may be used to visualize the thymus, intra-thoracic parathyroid tumor, lymph nodes, and the outer wall of the esophagus. Air is injected retrosternally. The patient should be told to expect his neck to become puffy and "crackle" as the air is absorbed into tissues. This is harmless and transitory.

Arthrography

Contrast medium may be injected into joint spaces of the knee or shoulder and films taken to evaluate tears in the menisci, damaged cruciate ligaments or articular condyles, or injury to the musculo-tendenous cuff. The procedure is contraindicated when there is local sepsis or active arthritis.

REFERENCES

Egan, Robert L.: Mammography, *Amer. J. Nurs.*, **66**(1):108, 1966.

Etter, Lewis E.: "Glossary of Words and Phrases Used in Radiology and Nuclear Medicine," Charles C Thomas, Springfield, Ill., 1960.

Meschan, Isadore: "Atlas of Normal Radiographic Anatomy," 2d ed., Saunders, Philadelphia, 1959.

Morgan, K. Z., and J. E. Turner: "Principles of Radiation Protection," Wiley, New York, 1969.

Rummerfeld, P. S., and M. J. Rummerfeld: What You Should Know about Radiation Hazards, *Amer. J. Nurs.*, **70**:780–786, 1970.

Saxton, H. M., and Basil Strickland: "Practical Procedures in Diagnostic Radiology," Grune & Stratton, New York, 1972.

TWELVE

RADIONUCLIDE STUDIES

Radioactivity has been the subject of intensive study since Henri Becquerel's pioneering work in the late nineteenth century. The scientific excitement in response to Röntgen's discovery of the x-ray in 1895 gave impetus to Becquerel's work with uranium compounds, which he had observed to fluoresce when exposed to sunlight. In a sense, his discovery of the emission of radiation by uranium was serendipity. He had put a package wrapped in black paper and containing a photographic plate and a sample of uranium ore in a drawer because the weather was cloudy, and he could not proceed with experiments involving sunlight. On developing this plate some time later, he found that the image of the ore was as clear as that produced when the preparation was exposed to sunlight, establishing the fact that uranium ore was a source of radiation. In 1897, Marie and Pierre Curie isolated two new elements, polonium and radium, which had this same property of radiant energy. Analysis of this phenomenon led to the identification of three types of radiation: alpha, beta, and gamma. Alpha and beta radiation were found to be charged particles: gamma radiation, to be electromagnetic waves.

With additional information regarding the nature of radioactivity, it was found that stable, i.e., nonradioactive, elements could be made radioactive by bombardment with high-energy particles. Studies accelerated under the demands of modern warfare and the fission of uranium led to an abundance of artificially produced radioactive elements. A natural corollary was the introduction of radioactive elements in research on biologic processes, followed by their use in diagnosis and treatment of disease and the establishment of the specialties of nuclear medicine and radiation biophysics.

ATOMIC STRUCTURE

It will be recalled that the atom is made up of a nucleus, which consists of neutrons and protons (only simple hydrogen contains no neutrons), and of electrons arranged in shells around the nucleus. These building blocks of atoms differ from each other in their state of electric charge and relative weight. Neutrons, which are the heaviest particles, are neutral, i.e., have no electric charge. Protons, slightly lighter in weight, are positively charged and are equal in number to the electrons in the free states of the elements. The mass of a proton is 1.68×10^{-24} g, which is 1,840 times that of an electron.

It is the behavior of the electrons that determines the combining of the elements together to form compounds:

Atom + atom (or atoms) → molecule

The electrons are arranged around the nucleus in layers, or shells, each level having the maximum number of electrons it may contain. The outer shell's content of electrons is variable, and this gives the atom its chemical characteristics. This shell is also known as the valence shell.

It will be seen that powerful electric forces are inherent in the stability of atomic structure. There must be a delicate balance between the cohesive and repulsive forces to maintain stability. When this does not obtain, spontaneous emission of radiation occurs as the nucleus tries to return to a balanced position and achieve stability. This emission of radiant energy was discovered by Becquerel in 1896 in his work on uranium compounds. All natural elements of atomic number greater than 83 and mass number greater than 209 are unstable and, therefore, radioactive.

The atomic number refers to the number of protons in the nucleus. This number could be applied to electrons in the free state as well, since the two components (electron and proton) are equal in the uncombined forms of the atoms, but it is not so applied because the loss or gain of electrons is basic to chemical combination to form molecules. The atomic number also determines the position of elements in the *periodic table*, a classification and arrangement of elements according to their chemical characteristics. Thus, elements with the same number of electrons in the outermost shell are classified together. For example, fluorine, chlorine, bromine, and iodine are in period 3 and are classified as halides. One might say that halide is the family name of this group of elements.

The mass number of the atom refers to the total number of neutrons and protons. When chemical symbols are used, the atomic number is written as a subscript preceding the symbol, and the mass number is written as a superscript preceding the symbol. For example, carbon, with 6 electrons, and 6 protons and 8 neutrons, is written $^{14}_{6}C$. Inclusion of the mass number is important in identifying specific radionuclides within a given family of an element.

DEFINITION OF ISOTOPES

Isotopes of a given element are alike in their numbers of electrons and protons, but they differ from each other in their mass numbers. For example, there are three isotopes of hydrogen: ^{1}H, ^{2}H, and ^{3}H. They differ from each other in that ^{1}H has one proton and no neutrons; ^{2}H has one proton and one neutron; and ^{3}H has one proton and two neutrons. The word isotope is derived from two Greek words: "isos," meaning "same," and topos, meaning "place." This "same place" refers to the fact that the isotopes an element have the same position held in the periodic table. In their natural state, free elements are made up of a mixture of atoms of the same atomic number and chemical properties but varying atomic mass. From this, it can be seen why atomic weights are not whole numbers, as might be expected. For example, the atomic weight of nitrogen is 14.008 because naturally occuring nitrogen is made up of 99.635 percent ^{14}N and 0.365 percent ^{15}N.

RADIONUCLIDES

In the first years of its development, nuclear medicine used the term *radioisotope* to describe the material with which it is concerned. The preferred term is *radionuclide*. This is a more specific as well as descriptive term. A clue will be apparent in the fact that this specialty in medicine is *nuclear* medicine, i.e., having to do with the use of elements whose nuclei have special properties. These nuclear properties of radiation are what determine the opportunities and limitations of the field.

Adding the prefix "radio" indicates that the nucleus of the atom gives off radiation energy. Radionuclides occur naturally, as isotopes of stable elements and as primary elements such as radium. However, nuclear medicine had to await the development of the cyclotron, the fission of uranium-235, and the discovery of techniques for bombarding atoms with neutrons before enough radionuclides became available for widespread use in a variety of ways.

Forms of Radiation Emitted from Radionuclides

Three types of radiation are possible in radionuclides: alpha (a), beta (β), and gamma (γ). Alpha particles are the heaviest by mass, being composed of two protons and two neutrons. The beta particle is the product of transformation of a neutron into a proton and an electron. The electron is emitted as a beta particle. Often a gamma ray will be emitted at the same time as the beta particle.

This is an effort on the part of the nucleus of the atom to reach a stable state, since emission of a beta particle can leave the nucleus in an excited, i.e., energized, state. By releasing energy in the form of gamma radiation, the atom reaches a stable state. It will be recalled from the discussion of x-rays that gamma radiation is energy in the form of electromagnetic waves.

It is interesting to note the different ranges of alpha and beta particles. The particles are dependent upon the emission energy for their velocities. The alpha particle has a range of 3 to 8 cm in air and a few micrometers in tissue. The beta particles may have velocities of nearly 95 percent of the speed of light (186,000 miles/s). Their range is several meters in air and up to 10 mm in tissue. The rate of evolution of alpha and beta particles is spontaneous and constant in a given element and is not altered by physical changes such as temperature and pressure.

When radioactive disintegration takes place, the changes in the nucleus bring about decay of the element. In naturally occuring radioactive elements, the decay brings about changes in the nucleus that alter the element, transforming it into another one lower in the periodic classification. The example of the decay of uranium-238 to form thorium is as follows:

$$^{238}_{92}U \rightarrow {}^{234}_{90}Th + 2 \text{ alpha}$$

This is but one of the 12 to 14 decay steps after which ^{238}U ends as a stable isotope of lead. Radiophosphorus ($^{32}_{15}P$) decays into sulfur ($^{32}_{16}S$) by emission of a beta particle. The change in this case does not involve mass, but it increases the atomic number.

$$^{32}_{15}P \rightarrow {}^{32}_{16}S + \beta^{-}$$

Another significant and useful characteristic of radioactive disintegration is seen in some instances in which there is delay in emission of the gamma radiation from the parent nuclide. When this happens, the daughter nuclide is in the metastable, or isomeric, state. This is indicated by the use of the letter m. For example, molybdenum-99 ($^{99}_{42}Mo$) disintegrates to the metastable daughter nuclide technetium-99m ($^{99m}_{43}$Tc) and finally to stable technetium-99:

$$^{99}_{42}\text{Mo} \rightarrow {}^{99m}_{43}\text{Tc} + \beta^- \rightarrow {}^{99}_{43}\text{Te} + \gamma$$

Technetium is easily separated from molybdenum chemically and can be used to advantage clinically.

Artificial Radioactivity

By bombarding the stable nucleus of any element, neutrons and protons can be injected, altering the nucleus to an unstable and, therefore, radioactive, state, creating a radionuclide. Particles released by radioactive disintegration also are a source of radio-nuclides.

Half-life of Radionuclides and Radioactive Elements

The disintegration process in radioactivity is measured in time as the *half-life period.* The half-life is the length of time required for conversion of half a given weight of a radioactive element or radionuclide to its disintegration product. The term may be confusing, but it is a necessary one because radioactive disintegration, or decay, is a continuing process at a given rate. Each radioactive element or radionuclide has a definite and measurable half-life. Figure 12-1 shows the meaning of half-life in graphic form.

The half-lives of parent and daughter radionuclides usually differ significantly—a phenomenon that can be used to advantage in medicine. For example, when $^{99m}_{43}$Tc is administered, it becomes concentrated in the brain, and scans of the brain can be done. An advantage of this daughter radionuclide is that its half-life is on 6 h. This means that the patient will be exposed to radioactive emissions for a relatively short time only. However, the parent radionuclide, $^{99}_{42}$Mo, has a half-life of 67 h. This longer half-life allows $^{99}_{42}$Mo to be shipped without severe loss in radioactivity. At the time the organ scan is to be done, the $^{99m}_{43}$Tc part of the mixture is chemically separated and administered.

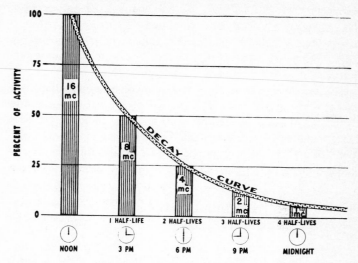

FIG. 12-1 The meaning of half-life. *(From Theodore Fields and Linton Seed, "Clinical Use of Radioisotopes: A Manual of Techniques," The Year Book Medical Publishers, Inc., Chicago, 1957, by permission of the publisher.)*

MEASUREMENT OF RADIOACTIVITY

A variety of measurements are applied to radioactivity, each of which concerns a specific function of the process. These are, generally speaking, quite technical and, since they are not necessary to the basic understanding of the practical measurement of radionuclide dosage, will not be discussed. The practical measurement of radionuclides is the Curie. The *Curie* (Ci) measures the disintegration process: one Curie equals 3.7×10^{10} disintegrations per second (dps), that is, the number of atoms of a given radioactive substance that disintegrate per second. The *millicurie* (mCi) equals 3.7×10^{7} dps. The *microcurie* (μCi) equals 3.7×10^{4} dps.

Calculations of half-life are essential in establishing the potency of radionuclides on arrival from the supplier, in timing the placement of orders, in calculating the results of tests, and in determining the amount of radioactivity in patients who have had therapeutic doses of radionuclides. Regulations governing use of radionuclides require that any patient who has 20 mCi or more of radionuclide in his body be hospitalized.

Everyone is subject to a certain amount of radiation energy under normal or usual circumstances. This comes from several sources. Cosmic rays account for an appreciable amount, and, as may be expected, the dose is twice as much at an elevation of 1 mile as it is at sea level. The average of the natural exposures has been estimated at between 100 and 200 millirads per year (rad = radiation absorption dose). These natural sources of radiation account for the background counts obtained as part of any examination measuring radioactivity.

MEASUREMENT OF RADIOACTIVITY IN PATIENTS AND MATERIALS

When radionuclides are used in diagnosis and treatment, measurements of the localization of the radionuclide, such as radioiodine in thyroid, and excretion of the material are made by various kinds of counters. These devices are designed to pick up the radiation and, by various means, show the actual count of radioactive emissions. With this information, the exact concentration in each area is calculated. Not only is this important in determining the diagnosis, but it is essential in disposing of waste materials that are also radioactive as well as in processing linens, etc. that have been rendered radioactive by use by the patient following treatment with radionuclides. The counting devices are constructed to take advantage of the fact that radioactive emissions ionize air, i.e., make electrical changes noted by alterations in electric charge. The information thus obtained is recorded in various ways, such as by actual count or by transforming the effect of the radioactive emissions on the counter to a recording device such as the scintiscanner (Fig. 12-2). In testing materials such as urine and blood, the well type of counter is used. Portable counters are used to monitor rooms and patient equipment subject to radioactivity.

Dual rectilinear scanners make it possible to scan from two different positions simultaneously. Another type of instrument in common use is the scintillation camera. This combines a scanner

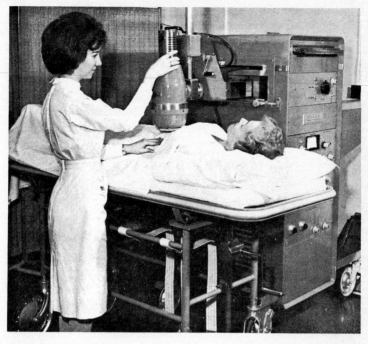

FIG. 12-2 Scintillation photoscanner used to scan small and large organs.
*(Courtesy of the Department of Nuclear Medicine, St. Mary's Hospital, St.
Louis, Mo.)*

with a camera which records the entire field from one position
rather than scanning line by line. Various types of scintillation
cameras are used, the differences being in the types of detectors
and image intensifiers.

EFFECTS OF RADIATION

As indicated in the discussion of radiology, radiation is powerful energy, which affects living tissue adversely by virtue of the
ionizing changes in cellular components. It can kill the cell or
alter its genetic apparatus. Judicious and discriminating use of this
tool in medicine is absolutely imperative. It must be treated with

the profound respect demanded by any powerful force with ability to kill.

General factors which are involved in potential for change due to radiation include the following:

1. Sensitivity to change.
2. Quantity of radiation.
3. Rate at which it is received (i.e., in intervals or single exposure).
4. Extent of the body exposed.
5. Part of the body exposed. (For example, it is more severe when it is delivered to the upper abdomen.)
6. Age of the individual — the more immature, the more sensitive.
7. Biologic variations among individuals.

Thus it can be seen that treatment with radiation is a complex matter, requiring the specialist in nuclear medicine or radiology to take many elements into consideration.

REGULATIONS GOVERNING USE OF RADIONUCLIDES

Recognizing the potential of radiation, the Atomic Energy Commission, in its roles of principal supplier and governing body, has set up regulations for the use and care of radioactive materials. They are designed to provide guidelines for medical personnel based on clinical radionuclide experience and practice.

When an institution or physician wants to carry out procedures involving radionuclides, an application for a license is made to the Atomic Energy Commission. Only those institutions or persons that have proper equipment and experienced personnel are considered. The physician must be specifically trained and experienced in the use of radionuclides. Institutional licenses are granted when facilities and personnel qualify in ability and training to carry out such a program, and the institution must have a medical radionuclides committee to review the use of radionuclides in research, diagnosis, and treatment.

The physician working with radionuclides is required to have a working knowledge of the principles and practices of radiologic health safety, of the use of instruments, of the mathematics basic to use and measurement of radioactivity, and of the biologic effects of radiation as well as experience in the actual use of radionuclides.

The International Commission on Radiological Protection (ICRP) provides guidance for standards of safety based on periodic study recommendations in all aspects of radiation risk.

RADIONUCLIDES IN DIAGNOSIS

Tracers

RADIOIODINE

A major resource in nuclear medicine, ^{131}I is one of 22 radionuclides of this element, ^{127}I being the stable form. Each has a different half-life, ranging from seconds to years. The half-life of ^{131}I is 8 days. ^{131}I is used both by itself and in combinations such as human serum albumin ($[^{131}I]$ HSA); it is also used in tagging reagents used in radioimmunoassay procedures. Classic examples of tagging physiologic compounds are tri-iodothyronine (T_3), and thyroxin (T_4), which allow for in vitro testing of thyroid function.

One of the tests of thyroid function using ^{131}I is the iodine-uptake test. In this test, the thyroid area is checked at intervals after administration of the tracer dose of ^{131}I to measure the amount of the radionuclide trapped by the thyroid gland, using the scintiscanner or scintillation camera (see Fig. 12-3). The uptake test is accompanied by measuring all urine excreted in 24 h following administration of the tracer dose and testing with the counter for the exact amount of radioiodine excreted. In euthyroid conditions, excretion is complete in 24 h; whereas in hyperthyroid conditions less time, and in hypothyroid conditions, more time, is needed by the body to clear the maximal amount of radioiodine by urinary excretion. Radioiodine uptake is inhibited by a number of factors. These include medication with Lugol's solution, treatment of the thyroid by x-rays, and medication with desiccated thyroid. In order that the radioiodine test be valid, therefore, any

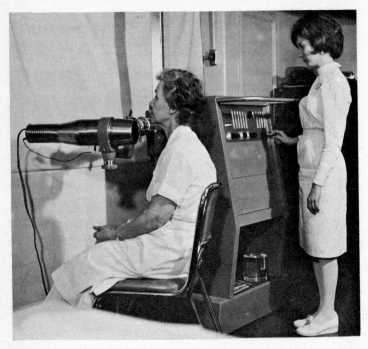

FIG. 12-3 Scintillation probe and scaler being used for measuring thyroid uptake of [131]I. *(Courtesy of the Department of Nuclear Medicine, St. Mary's Hospital, St. Louis, Mo.)*

such treatments must be discontinued for appropriate times before the radioiodine-uptake test is performed.

Radioiodine clearance from the blood by the thyroid may be tested. In this test, the amount of ^{131}I in the plasma is calculated at given intervals to determine how many milliliters of plasma are cleared, i.e., lose ^{131}I to the thyroid gland, per minute. Normally, the rate is 8 to 38 ml/min. In thyrotoxicosis, as much as 198 to 13,000 ml/min may be cleared.

The ratio of ^{131}I free in the plasma to that bound to blood protein may also be determined. In normal thyroid function, this ratio is found to be 0.30. (This figure is determined by dividing the free ^{131}I concentration by the protein-bound ^{131}I concentration.) A higher value indicates hyperthyroidism.

Refinements of diagnosis may be had by combining ^{131}I uptake and thyroid-stimulating hormone (TSH). A preliminary ^{131}I uptake test is made, and after administration of TSH, a second tracer dose is given to determine the response of the thyroid to this stimulation specific for it. In struma lymphomatosa, for example, there is no increased uptake; whereas there is an increase in cancerous and nodular goiter conditions.

Profiles of the thyroid are obtained by use of the scintiscanner or scintillation camera following a tracer dose of ^{131}I (Fig. 12-4). The profile reveals not only the extent of the thyroid gland but also the areas within it that are most active. These findings are valuable in both diagnosis and preparation for surgical procedures because they provide a map of the gland and the areas that require special attention. The in vitro T_3 and T_4 tests are described in Chapter 5.

RADIOCHROMIUM

The principal uses of radiochromium (^{51}Cr) are in studies of red blood cell survival and in determination of blood volume. Under proper conditions of pH, temperature, and time of incubation, nearly 90 percent of the tracer dose may be affixed to the cell content of blood. Sodium chromate readily binds with the protein of hemoglobin, but it does not participate in the metabolic processes of the red cells, and thus it is especially useful in these studies. Radiochromium is used in the differential diagnosis of anemias. For example, the normal half-life of the red cells is 27 to 86 days, but in hemolytic anemias this is reduced to 6 to 12 days. Thus, hemolytic anemias may readily be diagnosed by use of red blood cells tagged with radiochromium, since its half-life is 77.8 days.

To determine red blood cell mass and plasma volumes, blood from the patient is treated, under sterile conditions, with sodium chromate ($Na_2{}^{51}CrO_4$) and then injected into the patient. At given intervals, samples of blood are obtained, hematocrit values are determined, and the radioactivity of the plasma and whole blood is measured. With this information, the total volume of red blood

RADIOISOTOPES

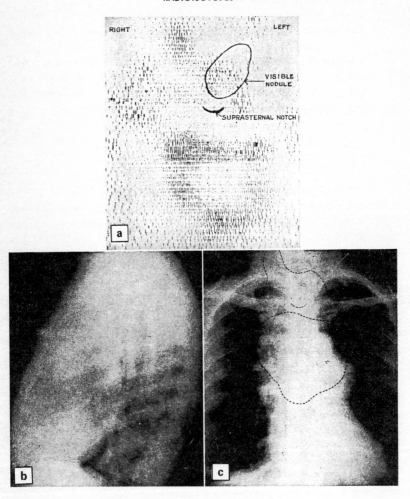

FIG. 12-4 A thyroid "map." *(From W. H. Beierwaltes, Philip C. Johnson, and Arthur J. Solari, "Clinical Use of Radioisotopes," W. B. Saunders Company, Philadelphia, 1957, by permission of the authors and publisher.)*

cells and whole blood is calculated. These tests are based on the fact that total volume may be determined by finding the degree of dilution or, as in this case, the radioactivity, of a solution when it is mixed with an unknown volume of another solution.

The same dilution technique is employed when ^{51}Cr is used to determine the actual volume of an exudate or transudate. The technique involves injection of a known amount of solution of sodium radiochromate into the site of the fluid accumulation and, after allowing time for mixture, withdrawing a sample of the fluid to count the radioactivity.

RADIOPHOSPHORUS

Since phosphorus is ubiquitous in the body, it is readily assimilated when injected into the body. Bony tissue contains more phosphorus than any other tissue. Phosphorus is utilized by cells in their process of metabolism and is contained in high proportion in the nuclei of cells. When the nuclei are multiplying at a rapid rate, and when, as in malignant conditions, they are large, the demand for phosphorus by the cells is high and rapid, and high concentration of the element is noted in such tissues.

RADIOCOBALT

Vitamin B_{12}, cyanocobalamin, may be tagged with ^{57}Co in order to follow its metabolic activity. It is especially valuable in the diagnosis of pernicious anemia. In this disease, lack of the intrinsic factor (the antianemic factor secreted by the stomach) leads to impaired absorption of vitamin B_{12}. The test involves giving the patient an oral tracer dose of ^{57}Co-tagged vitamin B_{12} and measuring its excretion. If absorption of vitamin B_{12} is impaired, the tagged vitamin is excreted in the stool. A dose of 0.5 g carmine red may also be given the patient when the vitamin is administered; when the dye appears in the stool, the test is completed.

In order to rule out the possibility that faulty B_{12} absorption is due to a different disease (such as sprue, pancreatic insufficiency, myxedema, or liver disease), an initial absorption test with low results may be followed by another test in which the injection of intrinsic factor and another oral tracer dose of the tagged vitamin are combined. If pernicious anemia is the problem, enhanced absorption should follow this treatment. In pernicious anemia, 70 to 100 percent of the vitamin will be excreted in about 4 days if no intrinsic factor is given. After the intrinsic factor is given, only 25 to 60 percent will be excreted.

The diagnostic test for pernicious anemia that is given the most often is the Schilling test. In this procedure, the urine, rather than the stools, is analyzed for ^{57}Co-tagged B_{12}. The test relies on the fact that, if the body is flooded with large parenteral doses of the vitamin, it will be excreted by the kidneys. (Under normal circumstances B_{12} is not found in the urine.)

The patient is given ^{57}Co-tagged B_{12} by mouth. This is followed by injection of 1,000 μg nonradioactive B_{12}. The patient saves all urine voided in the ensuing 24 h. If the patient is able to absorb B_{12}, the ^{57}Co-tagged vitamin will be found in the urine along with untagged vitamin.

RADIOIRON

Radioiron (^{59}Fe) is used to detect certain anemias. Iron is normally stored in the body for reuse by the hematopoietic system. When this storage and the relationship between the hemoglobin breakdown and synthesis of hemoglobin is disturbed, anemia results. In iron-deficiency anemias, the body's store of iron is low. In hemochromatosis, it is abnormally high and appears in cells that are not normally storage depots. In bone-marrow dysfunction, the iron store tends to be normal, but the synthesis of hemoglobin is blocked. In hemolytic anemias, there is a rapid breakdown and synthesis process. After injection of ^{59}Fe, the disappearance and subsequent reappearance of the nuclide in the peripheral circulation gives an indication of the rate of turnover in iron utilization. The test is most valuable in diagnosis of aplastic anemias.

Organ Scans

In addition to the previously discussed techniques of scanning the thyroid gland, materials have been synthesized using radionuclides in their structure which make possible the scanning of other major organs. These include the kidneys, brain, liver, lungs, pericardium, and bone lesions (see Fig. 12-5).

KIDNEYS

To scan the kidneys, the tagged diuretic ^{197}Hg-chlormerodrin (Neohydrin) is given intravenously, and the kidney areas are scanned after the drug has been concentrated in the kidneys (see Fig. 12-6a). There is no special preparation of the patient; the test requires from 1 to 3 h to complete. This type of scan is especially valuable from the patient's point of view, since no pressure or injection (e.g., retrograde pyelogram), trauma, or discomfort is involved. Space-occupying lesions such as cysts, abscesses, etc. appear as inactive (i.e., no concentration of the mercurial chlormerodrin) areas (see Fig. 12-6b).

In addition to scans, which provide information about structure, radionuclide studies related to renal functions of plasma clearance and excretion may be performed. The ^{131}I-sodium iodohippurate renogram provides information about the plasma clearance (filtration by the glomeruli), since iodohippurate is not bound by plasma proteins and readily passes through the glomerulur membrane. Chlormerodrin, on the other hand, is bound to proteins and requires removal by the renal tubules, thus reflecting the excretion capacity of the kidneys.

BRAIN

Iodinated human serum albumin ($[^{131}I]$ HSA) and ^{197}Hg-chlormerodrin have been used for brain scans, but since they present some disadvantages, sodium pertechnate-^{99m}Tc is being used with increasing frequency. The half-life of 6h and absence of β radiation in ^{99m}Tc are of particular

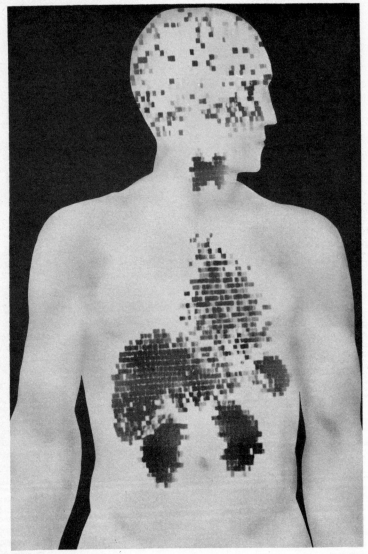

FIG. 12-5 Schematic representation of organs scanned by radioisotope techniques. Bone may also be scanned. *(Courtesy of the Department of Nuclear Medicine, Johns Hopkins Hospital, Baltimore, Md.)*

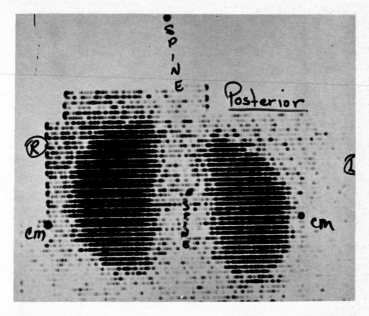

FIG. 12-6a Normal renal scan. Note that radioisotope material is concentrated by normal issue. *(Courtesy of the Department of Nuclear Medicine, St. Mary's Hospital, St. Louis, Mo.)*

advantage. In addition, less time is required for the scans (about 10 min per view, as compared to the 25 min required for ^{197}Hg-chlormerodrin). Scans are done in the anteroposterior and lateral positions to aid in localizing lesions. Brain tumors and certain vascular lesions are diagnosed by virtue of the fact that these lesions concentrate the scanning agents, resulting in a distinct area of darkening at their sites (see Fig. 12-7b). Good contrast is required, since there is normal concentration of the scanning agent in the venous sinuses, nasophrygeal mucosa, and scalp (see Fig. 12-7a).

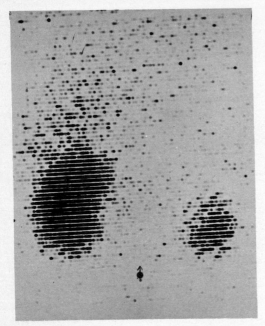

FIG. 12-6b Abnormal renal scan. Note that the left kidney is much smaller than the right, indicating nonfunctioning upper portion of the left kidney because of infarction. *(Courtesy of the Department of Nuclear Medicine, St. Mary's Hospital, St. Louis, Mo.)*

LIVER

The scanning agents of choice for liver scans are ^{131}I-rose bengal dye, [198]Au (gold) colloid, and ^{99m}Tc colloid. These materials are concentrated by normal liver cells, providing scan patterns that are darkest in areas of functioning hepatic tissue. The patterns seen in cirrhosis and hepatitis are mottled, the extent depending upon the amount of hepatocellular damage. The liver scan can be important in delineating the site for obtaining biopsy specimens (see Figs. 12-8*a* and *b*).

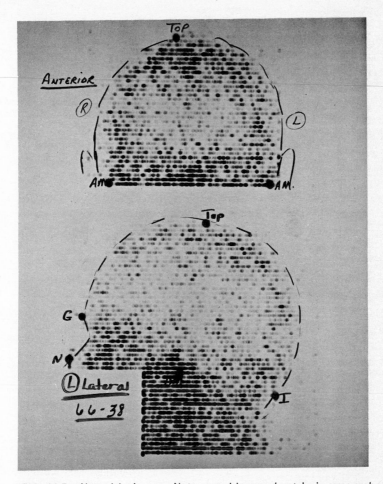

FIG. 12-7a Normal brain scan. Note normal increased uptake in areas such as venous sinuses, nasopharyngeal mucosa, and scalp. *(Courtesy of the Department of Nuclear Medicine, St. Mary's Hospital, St. Louis, Mo.)*

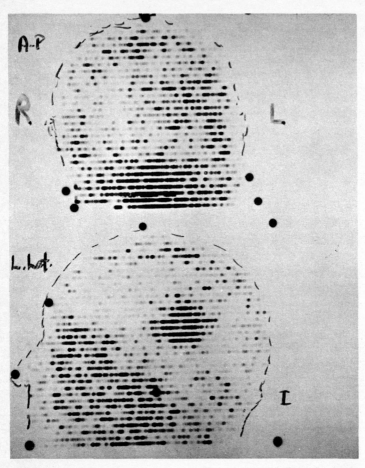

FIG. 12-7b   Abnormal brain scan. Note large density seen in the left temporal area resulting from increased uptake by abnormal tissue. *(Courtesy of the Department of Nuclear Medicine, St. Mary's Hospital, St. Louis, Mo.)*

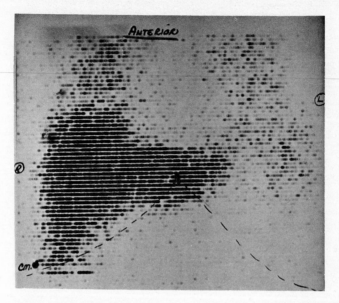

FIG. 12-8a Normal liver scan. The reticuloendothelial portions of the liver are seen, as well as small portions of the pulmonary area. Uptake in the left upper quadrant is the spleen. Note that normal tissue concentrates the radioisotopes. *(Courtesy of the Department of Nuclear Medicine, St. Mary's Hospital, St. Louis, Mo.)*

SPLEEN

Spleen scans are done using the colloids of ^{198}Au or ^{99m}Tc, the amount concentrated being considerably less than the amount that is concentrated by the liver. The scanning instrument must be adjusted to compensate for the difference in radioactivity. Structural aspects of the spleen and its location are the principal assessments to be made from the scan.

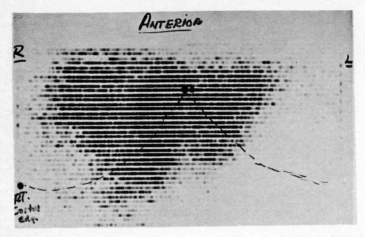

FIG. 12-8b Abnormal liver scan. Note the defect in the right lobe (absence of concentration) which extends below the costal margin, resulting from metastatic carcinoma. *(Courtesy of the Department of Nuclear Medicine, St. Mary's Hospital, St. Louis, Mo.)*

LUNG

Lung scans are of particular use in the differential diagnosis of pulmonary emboli, being both safe and simple, as well as definitive. Perfusion of the lung fields is accomplished when the scanning agent is introduced intravenously, as with macroaggregated [131I] HSA. Introduction of the radionuclide material by aerosol permits study of ventilation. In this technique, a mist of [131I] HSA, or the inert gas 133Xe (xenon) may be used. It is important to provide appropriate protection of the personnel when the inhalation route is used, lest accumulated exposure occur.

PERICARDIUM

The pericardium may be scanned using [131I] HSA, beginning the scan within 20 min after injection of the material. To demonstrate pericardial effusion or thickening, the scan is superimposed over a regular chest radiograph, and differences in the heart shadow outline are measured. In effusion (or more rarely, thickening), this difference is more than 1 cm.

BONE

Radionuclide scanning of bone has the distinct advantage of capability to visualize lesions as much as 6 months before changes are detectable in roentgenograms and a higher percent (95 percent) of detection of neoplastic disease. Various radionuclides may be used, such as ^{85}Sr, ^{87m}Sr, and ^{99m}Tc, with technetium becoming the one of choice. These materials are concentrated in areas of osteoblastic activity involved in the exchange of calcium. In bone malignancies, this activity is accelerated, concentrating the radionuclide in greater amounts than in the normal bone tissue.

REFERENCES

Beierwaltes, W. H., Philip C. Johnson, and A. J. Solari: "Clinical Use of Radioisotopes," Saunders, Philadelphia, 1957.

Fields, T., and L. Seed: "Clinical Use of Radioisotopes, "A Manual of Technique," 2d ed., Year Book, Chicago, 1963.

Morgan, K. Z., and J. E. Turner: "Principles of Radiation Protection," Wiley, New York, 1969.

Powsner, E. R., and D. E. Raeside: "Diagnostic Nuclear Medicine," Grune & Stratton, New York, 1971.

Sodee, D. Bruce, and Paul J. Early: "Technology and Interpretation of Nuclear Medicine Procedures," Mosby, St. Louis, 1972.

GLOSSARY

Acetest, a commercial preparation for testing for ketones in urine.

ac phos (acid phosphatase), an enzyme with optimal function at acid pH.

adenovirus, a DNA-containing virus associated with the common cold and implicated in oncogenesis. At least 28 types of adenovirus have been identified.

agglutinin, an antibody that causes clumping of the invading organism or cell.

agglutinogen, the substance contained in or on the red blood cell which determines the blood group of the cells; also referred to as factor, gene, or antigen.

alb (albumin), one of the blood proteins.

aliquot, a small measured portion of a given solution.

alk phos (alkaline phosphatase), an enzyme with optimal function in an alkaline medium.

alpha particle, helium nucleus (two protons and two neutrons) with a double positive charge.

amm N (ammonia nitrogen), the nitrogen portion of the molecule. Also abbreviated NH_4^+.

amniocentesis, removal of fluid from the amniotic sac of the pregnant uterus.

ANA (antinuclear antibody), a test for lupus erythematosus.

anion, a negatively charged ion. When NaCl ionizes, the chloride becomes an anion.

anisocytosis, variation in the size of red blood cells.

anode, the positive pole of an electrical system. Negatively charged particles (anions) are attracted to the anode.

antibody, a substance produced by the body in response to a protein or proteinlike substance foreign to the body.

antigen, a protein or proteinlike substance that can incite production of antibody when introduced into the body.

arbovirus, an RNA-containing virus which is arthropod-borne and causes encephalitis.

assay, analysis of a compound or a body fluid for the presence and amount of a given substance (particularly in testing for hormones).

ASTO (antistreptolysin O), the antibody to a substance elaborated by some streptococci.

atomic number, the number of protons in the nucleus. Also, the number of electrons outside the nucleus of a neutral atom.

^{198}**Au,** radionuclide of gold.

autosome, a chromosome other than the sex chromosomes. There are 22 pairs of autosomes and one pair of sex chromosomes in the human cell.

bacteriophage, a virus specifically parasitic to a bacterial species; used particularly in studies of staphylococci speciation.

basophilia, in hematology, a bluish tinge in the red blood cells. It may be stippled or diffuse.

beta particle, an atomic particle having the mass and charge of an electron which may be emitted (β^-) or captured (β^+) by the nucleus of an atom.

bronchography, study of the bronchial tree by radiographs after instillation of a radiopaque medium.

BSP (bromsulfalein), a dye administered in the study of liver function.

buffer, a weak acid and a salt of that acid in solution, the combination of which maintains the pH of a solution at a given level despite the addition of hydrogen or hydroxyl ions.

buffy coat, the layer of white blood cells seen lying on top of the layer of red blood cells when unclotted blood is centrifuged.

BUN (blood urea nitrogen), the nitrogen fraction of urea.

Ca, calcium.

carboxyhemoglobin, carbon monoxide combined with hemoglobin.

cardioangiography, radiologic study of the heart and great vessels with use of radiopaque medium.

cassette, the x-ray film holder.

casts, molds of tubules or bronchi. The former are composed of precipitated protein, the latter of mucus and cells.

cathode, the negative pole of an electrical system. Positively charged particles (cations) are attracted to the cathode.

cation, a positively charged ion. When NaCl ionizes, sodium is the cation.

CBC (complete blood count), comprised of hemoglobin, red blood cell count (or hematocrit), white blood cell count, and differential count.

CEA (carcinoembryonic antigen), a glycoprotein of the glycocalyx secreted by gastrointestinal cells. Elevations of the blood level of CEA are associated with some malignancies, various nonmalignant but inflammatory diseases, and surgical trauma.

ceruloplasmin, a blood protein containing copper.

chlormerodrin, a contrast medium (Neohydrin) used in radiography of the renal system.

chol (cholesterol), an alcohol associated with fats.

cholangiography, radiologic examination of the biliary tree with use of radiopaque medium.

cholecystography, radiologic examination of the gallbladder with use of a radiopaque medium.

cineradiography, motion-picture studies with x-ray exposures.

Cl, chlorine or chloride ion.

Clinistix, a commercial product for testing urine for albumin.

Clinitest, a commercial product for testing urine for glucose.

coagulopathy, abnormal coagulation of the blood.

CO_2 combining power (carbon dioxide combining power), the capacity of the plasma to take up carbon dioxide.

colloidal solution, a suspension of very small particles, which do not settle out of solution but are not dissolved in it.

compatibility, in immunohematology, a satisfactory cross match between donor and recipient bloods.

complement, a protein substance in the blood of all animals which is an essential element in antigen-antibody reaction.

complement fixation, using up, or binding, of complement in a serologic determination.

contrast medium, a liquid or semisolid material used to visualize body cavities and structures in radiologic examinations. These contrast media are radiopaque.

Coombs' test, a test for incomplete, or coating, antibodies. Direct: a test of the red blood cells for coating with this type of antibody. Indirect: a test of serum for the presence of unattached incomplete antibodies, particularly in anti-Rh titers and cross matches.

corpus hemorrhagicum, a hemorrhagic body on the surface of the ovary.

corpus luteum, a yellowish body on the surface of the ovary, formed at the release site after the release of an ovum.

CPK (creatine phosphokinase), an enzyme essential to the phosphorylation of creatine, found particularly in muscle tissue.

^{51}**Cr,** radionuclide of chromium.

creat (creatinine), a nitrogenous compound formed in the breakdown of creatine and excreted in urine.

CRPA (C-reactive protein agglutination), test used to evaluate inflammatory diseases.

cryoprecipitate, plasma protein fraction containing antihemophilic globulin.

CSF, cerebrospinal fluid.

cyanocobalamin, vitamin B_{12}. Radiocobalt-cyanocobalamin is used in the Schilling test.

cytolysin, an antibody or agent that breaks down cells.

Curie, a measurement of radioactivity (3.7×10^{10} disintegrations/ sec). Named for Marie and Pierre Curie, discoverers of radium. Abbreviated Ci.

daughter nuclide, an intermediate radioactive disintegration product of a precursor radionuclide.

deciliter, 1/10 liter. Abbreviated dl.

Dextrostix, a commercial product used for rough quantitative estimates of glucose.

Diagnex, a commercial product used to detect the presence of gastric acidity. Used as a screening test.

DIC (disseminated intravascular coagulation), abnormal coagulation resulting in exhaustion of certain coagulation factors leading to a bleeding syndrome.

dilution, serial, dilution of a substance such as serum by a series of mixtures of serum and diluent, each tube increasing the dilution sequentially.

Eaton agent, etiologic agent of primary atypical pneumonia, also known as PPLO (one of the Mycoplasmas).

EDTA (ethylenediaminetetraacetic acid), also known as sequestrene, an anticoagulant for blood specimens.

electrode, a pole of an electrical system.

electrolyte, a compound that dissociates into ions when dissolved in water, thus rendering the solution capable of conducting electricity.

electron, a negatively charged particle of mass 0.0005488 mass unit and in orbit about the nucleus of an atom.

electrophoresis, separation of serum proteins by electric current.

equivalent, in chemistry the weight of an element or radical that will combine with one gram molecular weight of hydrogen or oxygen.

erythrocyte, a red blood cell.

exfoliative cytology, study of epithelial cells that have sloughed off.

exudate, an accumulation of fluid as a result of an inflammatory process.

^{59}**Fe,** radioactive isotope of iron.

fib (fibrinogen), a plasma protein essential to the formation of a clot (fibrin).

fibrin split products, fractions of fibrin resulting from lysis of clots.

filter, in radiology, plates of copper and/or aluminum used to remove or lessen the effect of secondary radiation.

flagellum, threadlike projection from a bacterium or protozoan, which serves as a means of locomotion.

flocculation, the fine clumping seen in certain antigen-antibody reactions.

fluorescent antibody, an antibody tagged with a fluorescein dye to make it glow under fluorescent light.

fluoroscopy, radiologic study with use of a fluorescent screen rather than film.

Friedman test, a test for pregnancy with rabbit as test animal.

frog test, a test for pregnancy with male frog as test animal.

Galatest, a commercial product for testing urine for glucose.

galvanometer, an instrument used to detect the intensity and/or direction of electric current.

gamma radiation, electromagnetic waves, measured in millielectron volts.

glob (globulin), a blood plasma or serum protein.

gram-negative, those bacterial organisms which take up the red dye of Gram's stain.

gram-positive, those bacterial organisms which take up the deep purple dye of Gram's stain.

Guthrie test, a screening test for elevated levels of phenylalanine in the blood.

half-life, the length of time required for one-half the radioactivity to decay.

Hanger's test, cephalin flocculation test, a test of liver function.

Hct (hematocrit), a measurement of the proportion of the blood cells after centrifugation, particularly the red blood cells.

hemagglutinin, an antibody that causes red blood cells to clump together.

hemagglutinin inhibition, prevention of clumping of red blood cells.

hemoglobinemia, free hemoglobin present in the blood serum or plasma.

hemoglobinuria, free hemoglobin present in the urine.

hemolysin, an antibody that causes the red blood cells to break down.

hemolysis, breakdown of red blood cells. Alpha hemolysis: the effect of a group of streptococci and some pneumococci, which produce a green zone around the colonies of the organisms growing on blood agar. Beta hemolysis: the effect of certain species of bacteria, which produce a clear zone around the colonies of the organisms growing on blood agar.

hemophilia A, classic hemophilia in which there is a deficiency of antihemophilic globulin. It occurs most frequently in males and is generally carried by females.

hemophilia B, a bleeding disorder due to deficiency in plasma thromboplastin component; occurs most frequently in males. Also known as Christmas disease.

hemophilia C, a bleeding disorder due to deficiency in plasma thromboplastin antecedent which occurs in both sexes.

hemostasis, the dynamic factors involved in maintaining balance between free-flowing blood and coagulation, including the ability of the capillaries to restrict blood flow from injured sites.

heterophile, interspecies reaction of agglutination of red blood cells. It is used particularly in testing for infectious mononucleosis.

heterozygous, of differing genetic characteristics with regard to a given quality.

Hgb (hemoglobin), the red-colored respiratory pigment present in the red blood cells.

HLA (human lymphocyte antibody), used in pretransplant screening tests.

^{131}I, a radionuclide of iodine.

IgA, IgD, IgE, IgG, IgM, fractions of immunoglobulin.

ICRP, International Commission on Radiation Protection.

$[^{131}I]$ **HSA,** human serum albumin tagged with radioiodine.

immune bodies, the antibodies produced in response to a protein foreign to the body.

immunohematology, the study of blood groups and factors, sensitizations between factors, and blood banking.

inverse proportion, a relationship between two variables by which, as one is increased numerically, the other is decreased at the same time.

ion, an atomic particle, atom, or chemical radical with a positive or negative electric charge.

ionization, the change in a neutral atom or molecule when it acquires an electric charge.

iron-binding capacity, the ability of the blood protein, transferrin, to bind and transport iron. Abbreviated TIBC (total iron-binding capacity).

isohemagglutination, clumping of the red blood cells of one individual by the serum of another individual of the same species.

isozyme, an enzyme in a given "family" function (e.g., lactic acid dehydrogenase) but differing in organ specificity.

karyotype, identification of chromosome patterns using cell cultures.

kernicterus, staining of the cells of the brain with bilirubin when it is present in greatly elevated levels in the newborn infant.

ketosteroid, a hormone characterized by the presence of a ketone radical.

Kolmer test, a complement-fixation test for syphilis.

lactic acid dehydrogenase, an enzyme essential to the metabolism of lactic acid. Abbreviated LDH.

larvae, immature forms of certain parasites. There are two forms: rhabdite and filariform. Rhabdite forms are intermediary and are noninfective. Filariform forms, the next step in maturation, are the infective forms.

LE cell (lupus erythematosus cell), a neutrophilic leukocyte that has phagocytized chromatin material into its cytoplasm, seen in about 50 percent of cases of lupus erythematosus.

lipoprotein, lipids (triglycerides, cholesterol) bound to protein of blood.

macrocyte, a red blood cell larger in diameter than the upper limits of normal.

mammography, examination of breast tissue by radiologic means.

mass number, the number of protons and neutrons in the nucleus of the atom.

Master's two-step, an exercise used in electrocardiography to incite changes typical of angina pectoris.

MCH (mean corpuscular hemoglobin), average amount of hemoglobin per cell. Reported in picograms (10^{-12} g).

MCHC (mean corpuscular hemoglobin concentration), average amount of hemoglobin in 1 dl packed red cells. Reported in grams.

MCV (mean corpuscular volume), average size of red cells. Reported in cubic micrometers.

metastable, the state of a radionuclide in which the gamma ray is not emitted immediately after disintegration of the parent nuclide.

methemoglobin, decomposed hemoglobin.

microcyte, a red blood cell smaller in diameter than the lower limits of normal.

millicurie, a measure of radioactivity (1/1000 Curie). Abbreviated mCi.

milliequivalent, 1/1000 equivalent. Abbreviated meq.

milliosmol, 1/1000 osmol. Abbreviated mOsm.

milliroentgen, a measure of x-radiation (1/1000 roentgen). Abbreviated mr.

monoclonal, a cell-culture line derived from a single cell.

Mycoplasma, a very small microorganism which has bacterial properties but differs in the composition of the cell wall.

myelography, radiologic study of the spinal canal with use of radiopaque media.

myxovirus, an RNA-containing virus, e.g., influenza, parainfluenza, measles, and mumps.

neutralizing antibodies, substances that inhibit infection by viruses in test animals or tissue cultures. They are immune bodies.

neutron, an uncharged particle contained in the nucleus of an atom. Its mass is 1.00892 mass units.

opsonin, an antibody that causes invading bacteria to be more susceptible to phagocytosis.

osmol, the number of ions into which a molecule dissociates in solution; or the number of molecules of a nonionizable substance, multiplied by the osmotic coefficient. One osmol of any solution depresses the freezing point of the solution $1.86°C$.

osmolality, the functional relationship between the number of molecules or ions present in a solution and the effect on the boiling point, freezing point, and vapor pressure of the solution.

osmotic pressure, the pressure exerted when two solutions of different concentrations are separated by a membrane that is permeable to the solvent only.

oxidation, the combining of a substance with oxygen; the removal of electrons, by chemical means, from atoms or ions (*cf.* reduction).

oxyhemoglobin, hemoglobin combined with oxygen.

^{32}P, radionuclide of phosphorus.

P_{CO_2}, the partial pressure of carbon dioxide; carbon dioxide tension.

Papanicolaou stain, a special staining process used in exfoliative cytology.

papovavirus, a DNA-containing virus which causes wart formation.

PBI (protein-bound iodine), iodine that has been adsorbed by protein molecules in the blood.

pH, the hydrogen-ion concentration of a solution, i.e., its acidity or alkalinity.

phage typing, determination of the specific type of an organism; particularly used in studies of staphylococci (see bacteriophage).

phenylketone, any of several intermediate end products of amino acid metabolism, particularly phenylalanine, phenylpyruvic acid, and *o*-hydroxyphenylacetic acid.

pherogram, the pattern produced by separation of proteins by electric current.

photofluorography, in radiology, the process of taking a picture of a fluoroscopic image.

picornavirus, a group of RNA-containing viruses, among which are the polioviruses, Coxsackie viruses, ECHO viruses, and rhinoviruses.

planigraph, a series of radiographic films taken at multiple, sequential depths. Also called tomograph.

platelets, very small cells that are an essential element in the coagulation process. Also called thrombocytes.

pneumoencephalography, radiologic study of the subarachnoid space after injection of air into the space.

PO$_4$, phosphate ion.

piokilocytosis, variation from normal shade in red blood cells.

polyclonal, a cell-culture line derived from more than one cell.

postprandial, after a meal.

poxvirus, a group of DNA-containing viruses, among which are those causing smallpox and chickenpox.

PPLO (a pleuropneumonia-like organism), now considered to be a *Mycoplasma* and the etiologic agent of primary atypical pneumonia. Also known as Eaton agent.

precipitin, an antibody that causes a fine precipitation of foreign protein.

pro time (prothrombin time), a test for one of the elements involved in the coagulation process, used particularly in anticoagulant therapy to judge dosage.

proton, a positively charged particle contained in the nucleus of an atom, with mass 1.007593 mass units; also, the hydrogen ion.

PSP (phenolsulfonphthalein), a dye used in testing kidney function.

PTT (partial thromboplastin time), a test used in assessing defects in coagulation.

pyelography, radiologic study of the urinary system with use of radiopaque medium, which may be introduced by intravenous or retrograde methods.

qualitative, relating to the quality or kind of a given element or compound.

quantitative, relating to the quantity or amount of a given element or compound.

radiograph, an image produced by exposing the part of the body to x-rays and recording the exposure on special photographic film.

radiology, the study of, and practice of the use of, x-rays in medicine.

radionuclide, one of a group of atomic species having the same chemical properties and the same atomic number but different mass number, which emits beta particle(s) or gamma rays.

radiopaque, impervious to x-rays.

RBC (red blood cells), red blood cell count.

reduction, removal of oxygen from a compound chemically; also lowering of the positive charge of an ion or element.

refractive index, the amount of change of the pathway of light through a solution. It is a means of measuring total solids dissolved in a solvent.

renal threshold, the level of concentration in the blood above which a substance (glucose, for example) is excreted in the urine.

reovirus, an RNA-containing virus which causes respiratory and enteric disease.

rhinovirus, an RNA-containing virus associated with the common cold.

RIA (radioimmunoassay), a technique for quantifying materials present in the blood in minute amounts combining principles of immunology and nuclear medicine.

roentgen, a unit of measurement of x-radiation. Named for Wilhelm Konrad Rontgen (1845–1923), German physicist, who discovered x-ray. Abbreviated r.

roentgenogram, an image recorded on special photographic film by exposure to x-rays (*cf.* radiograph).

roentgenology, the study of, and practice of the use of, x-rays in medicine.

saprophyte, a microorganism that does not produce disease but may be found in or on the body.

Schilling test, a procedure used to determine the absorption of vitamin B_{12}.

Schwachman test, a screening test for the salt content of sweat, used in the diagnosis of cystic fibrosis.

scintillation, the flash of light produced when a particle from a radioactive material strikes a crystal detector.

scintillation camera, a device recording the emission of radioactivity, used in obtaining scans of organs, etc.

scintiscanner, an instrument used to detect the location and amount of radioactivity.

serology, the study of antigen-antibody reactions, particularly in reference to infectious agents.

SGOT (serum glutamic-oxaloacetic transaminase), an enzyme.

SGPT (serum glutamic-pyruvic transaminase), an enzyme.

SMA-12, sequential multiple analysis of 12 blood chemistry constituents.

specific gravity, the measurement of the amount of dissolved material in a liquid, using comparison with displacement of a mercury bulb as the index. Specific gravity is the weight of 1 ml of solution.

spirella, a group of microorganisms having loose, flexible coils.

spirochete, a group of microorganisms having tight, rigid coils.

spirometer, an instrument for measuring the amount of air taken into and expelled by the lungs, using a closed chamber with movable bell-like cover attached to a kymograph which plots the amount on a graph.

stippling, dotted forms seen in red blood cells. Basophilic stippling is bluish in color; Schuffner's stippling is reddish.

sulfhemoglobin, hemoglobin combined with sulfur instead of oxygen.

T_3 (tri-iodothyronine), a thyroid hormone with three iodine atoms.

T_4 (thyroxine), a thyroid hormone with four iodine atoms.

technitium, a chemical element related to molybdenum; ^{99m}Tc is the radionuclide of this element.

TGT (thromboplastin-generation time), a test used in assessing coagulation defects.

Thorn test, a test of adrenal capacity, utilizing total eosinophil counts.

thrombocyte, small cell in the blood, essential to blood coagulation. Also called platelet.

thromboplastin, a compound essential to coagulation of the blood.

thromboplastinogen, the precursor of thromboplastin.

thromboplastinogenase, the enzyme that activates the formation of thromboplastinogen.

titer, the highest dilution of a solution or serum that will produce a given reaction.

tomograph, a series of radiographs taken at multiple, sequential depths. Also called planigraph.

tot prot (total protein), the blood proteins: albumin, globulin, fibrinogen.

TPI *(Treponema pallidum* immobilization), a specific test for syphilis.

transudate, an accumulation of fluid in the body cavity secondary to stasis or noninflammatory disease.

ultrafiltration, removal of all but the very smallest particles.

Uristix, a commercial product used to test urine for glucose and protein.

Vacutainer, a system composed of needle, adapter, and tube from which air has been evacuated for obtaining blood by venipuncture.

van den Bergh's test, bilirubin test.

VDRL, flocculation test for syphilis.

ventriculography, radiologic study of the ventricles of the brain after introduction of a radiopaque medium or air.

WBC, white blood cell count.

xanthochromasia, yellow coloration, particularly used in describing the appearance of cerebrospinal fluid.

APPENDIX

Test	Material required	Special considerations
Acetone	Urine, plasma, serum	
Acid phosphatase	Serum	
Addis' count	Urine	12- or 24-h specimen
Albumin	Serum	Fasting specimen
	Urine	Random or 24-h specimen
Alcohol (ethanol)	Serum	Label time collected; use nonalcoholic antiseptic to cleanse puncture site
Alkaline phosphatase	Serum	
Amino acids	Urine, serum	
Ammonia nitrogen	Serum	
Amniotic-fluid analysis	Amniotic fluid	
Bilirubin		Protect from light
Enzymes		Maintain sterility

Test	Material required	Special considerations
Karyotype		Maintain sterility
Amphetamines	Serum, urine	
Amylase	Serum	
Antinuclear antibody	Serum	
Anti-streptococcus MG	Serum	
Arsenic	Serum, urine, hair and nail clippings	
Australia antigen (see HAA)	Serum	
Barbiturates	Serum, whole blood, urine	
Bence-Jones protein	Urine	Random sample
Bicarbonate	Plasma, serum	Exclude atmospheric air
Bile	Urine	
Bilirubin	Serum	Fasting specimen
	Urine	
	Amniotic fluid	Protect from light
	Stool	
Bleeding time		In vivo test
Blood type	Whole blood	
Bromides	Serum	
Bromsulfalein (BSP)	Serum	Fasting state
Brucella antibodies (undulant fever)	Serum	
Calcium	Serum	
	Urine	Random specimen for Sulkowitch; 24-h quantitative
Carboxyhemoglobin	Whole blood	
Catecholamines	Urine	Random or 24-h specimen, as directed
Cerebrospinal fluid	CSF	
Cell count		Perform immediately
Culture		Maintain sterility
Ceruloplasmin	Serum	
Chloride	Serum, plasma	Promptly remove serum or plasma from cells
Cholesterol	Serum	Fasting specimen
Cholinesterase	Serum	
Chorionic gonadotropin (pregnancy, etc.)	Serum	
	Urine	First morning, concentrated specimen

Test	Material required	Special considerations
Clearances		
Creatinine	Serum and urine	Paired specimens at timed
Urea		intervals
Inulin		
CO_2 combining power	Serum, plasma	Exclude atmospheric air
Coagulation-factor	Plasma	Minimal trauma in veni-
assays		puncture; two-syringe
		technique as directed
Coagulation time	Whole blood	
Cold agglutinins	Serum	Keep at room temperature
		or 37°C
Complement fixation	Serum	For virus and rickettsial
		studies, acute and con-
		valescent specimens
		required
Coombs'		
Direct	Whole blood	Frequently done on umbil-
		ical cord blood
Indirect	Serum	
Copper	Serum, plasma	
Coproporphyrins	Urine	Random or 24-h specimens,
		as directed; protect from
		light
Cortisol	Plasma	Label time collected
C-reactive protein	Serum	
Creatine phosphokinase	Serum	
Creatinine	Serum	
Cross match	Serum, cells	
Cryoglobulins	Serum	Maintain at 37°C
Diacetic acid	Urine	
Differential cell count	Blood smear	
Digitalis derivatives	Serum	Label derivative sought
Doriden (glutethimide)	Serum	
	Gastric lavage	
Electrophoresis	Serum	Fasting specimen
Eosinophil count	Whole blood	
Estrogens	Urine	24-h specimen
Febrile agglutinins	Serum	
(typhoid, paratyphoid,		
Weil-Felix)		
Fibrinogen	Plasma	

Test	Material required	Special considerations
Fishberg's concentration	Urine	Specimens as directed
Fluorescent *Treponema* antibodies (FTA)	Serum	
Galactose	Urine, whole blood	
Gastric analysis	Gastric contents	Fasting and after test meal
	Urine	In Diagnex blue test only
Globulins	Serum	
Glucose	Serum	As directed for time
	Urine	Random specimen
Glucose 6-phospho-dehydrogenase	Red blood cells	
Guthrie	Whole blood	May be collected on filter paper
Hemagglutinins	Serum	Acute and convalescent specimens
Hemoglobin	Whole blood	May be used for electrophoresis
	Serum	Avoid hemolysis
Hepatitis-associated antigen (HAA or HBAg)	Serum	
Heterophile antigen	Serum	
Homogentisic acid	Urine	
17-Hydroxycortico-steroids	Plasma	Test immediately or freeze
	Urine	24-h specimen, as directed
5-Hydroxyindoleacetic acid (5-HIAA)	Urine, qualitative	Random specimen
	Urine, quantitative	24-h specimen
Immunoglobulins	Serum	
Iron (total, binding capacity, saturation)	Serum	Avoid hemolysis
Ketone bodies	Urine, serum	
17-Ketosteroids	Urine	24-h specimen; refrigerate
Lactic acid dehydrogenase	Serum	Avoid hemolysis
Latex agglutination	Serum	
Lead	Whole blood	
	Urine	24-h specimen
Lipase	Serum	
Lipoproteins	Serum	At least 12-h fast
Lithium	Serum	
Macroglobulins	Serum	

Test	Material required	Special considerations
Methemoglobin	Whole blood	
Microscopic, urine	Sediment	Examine within 1 h
Neutralizing antibody	Serum	Maintain sterility
Osmolality	Serum, urine	
Osmotic fragility	Whole blood	
Oxygen (tension, content, saturation)	Serum, plasma	Exclude atmospheric air
pH	Serum, plasma	Label source (arterial or venous); exclude air; remove from cells quickly; notify laboratory before collecting specimen
Phenolsulfthalein excretion	Urine	As directed
Phosphates (phosphorus)	Serum	
Platelet count	Whole blood	
Porphyrins	Urine	Note time of collection; test immediately; protect from light
Potassium	Serum	Avoid hemolysis; remove from cells promptly
Pregnancy	Urine	Concentrated, first-morning specimen
	Serum	
Protein	Serum	Fasting specimen
	Urine	Random or 24-h specimen as directed
Prothrombin time	Plasma	Sodium citrate anticoagulant
Red blood cell count	Whole blood	
Reticulocyte count	Whole blood	
Rh factors	Whole blood	
Rheumatoid factor	Serum	
Sedimentation rate	Whole blood	
Seminal-fluid analysis	Seminal fluid	Maintain body temperature
Sodium	Serum	
Specific gravity	Urine	
Sulkowitch's	Urine	Random or 24-h specimen, as directed

Test	Material required	Special considerations
Thyroid hormones Thyroxine (T₄) Tri-iodothyronine (T₃) Thyroid-binding globulin (TBG)	Serum	
Treponema pallidum immobilization (TPI)	Serum	Maintain sterility
Triglycerides	Serum	At least 12-h fast
Tularemia antibodies (rabbit fever)	Serum	
Urea nitrogen	Serum	
Urobilinogen	Urine	May be 2-h timed specimen; perform test promptly; protect from light
Vanillylmandelic acid (VMA)	Urine	24-h specimen; no coffee or fruits 2 days prior to test
VDRL	Serum	
White blood cell count	Whole blood	
Widal	Serum	

INDEX